Most

MW00612563

The Science Behind Why You
Should Eat More Veggies

By Ahnjel Ali, LAc, DiplAc

Body Mind Spirit Publishing Group

Los Angeles, California

Mostly Vegan

ISBN 978-0-9856899-2-6

Library of Congress Control Number: 2021918028

Body Mind Spirit Publishing Group

Los Angeles, California

Other Books by Ahnjel Ali

Full Body 30 Day Vegan Cleanse
&
30 Easy Vegan Lunches to Bring
to Work

Cover Photo by Riley Ali

Edited by Terry Nozick

DEDICATION

First and foremost is my wonderful husband Majid
Ali. I thank you for taking this journey with me and
growing and having a great time along the way. You
have taught me so much and made my life richer.
My love for you just grows deeper.
Next is our two sons, Riley and Asher, I will never be
able to tell you enough how much I love you and
how grateful I am that you have been ours. Our lives
are so much richer and joyful because of you.

CONTENTS

INTENDED USE STATEMENT

The content of this book is intended for information purposes only. The medical information in this book is intended as general information only and should not be used in any way to diagnose, treat, cure, or prevent disease. The goal of the book is to present and highlight scientific information garnered through research. In so doing the intention is to show that research has seen a relationship between foods eaten and effects to the human body.

It is the sole responsibility of the reader of this book to comply with the direction of their personal physician.

DISCLAIMER AND NOTICES

The information provided in this book is not intended as a substitute for personalized medical advice, the reader of this book should comply with the advice given from his/her own licensed medical provider. It is left to the discretion of and is the sole responsibility of the reader to determine if eating more vegetables is appropriate for his/her health. The author and publisher cannot be held responsible for the information or any inadvertent errors or omissions of the information.

The information provided in this book is designed to provide helpful information on the subjects discussed. This book is not meant to be used, nor should it be used, to diagnose or treat any medical condition. For diagnosis or treatment of any medical problem, consult your own physician. The publisher and author are not responsible for any specific health or allergy needs that may require medical supervision and are not liable for any damages or negative consequences from any treatment, action, application or preparation, to any person reading or following the information in this book.

The information in this book should not be construed as a claim or representation that the vegetables written about will provide a specific cure, palliative or ameliorative. The nutritional information should be regarded as adjuvant measures to the recommendations of the readers own personal licensed medical provider.

The Food and Drug Administration has not evaluated the information in this book.

ABOUT AHNJEL ALI

Ahnjel Ali has been a Licensed Acupuncturist and Chinese Herbalist since 1993. Ahnjel is also Nationally Certified as an Acupuncturist and is certified as a Sports Nutritionist.

For a number of years, Ahnjel was an associate of Dr. Matt Van Benschoten, a ground-breaking Doctor of Chinese Medicine. It was while working with Dr. Van Benschoten that Ahnjel learned how to use herbs from a Western approach, developing an understanding of which herbs had anti-bacterial or anti-viral properties, which herbs had anti-inflammatory effects or hormonal effects, etc. This was a turning point for Ahnjel, where she began practicing in a way that bridged Eastern and Western Medicine. Now this would be termed Functional.

Ahnjel still practices in Los Angeles and has an herbal pharmacy with more than 300 individual herbs, allowing Ahnjel to treat patients with autoimmune disorders, all types of digestive disorders, hormonal imbalances, all types of headaches and migraines, as well as other health problems.

Acknowledgements

I feel very fortunate to have many people who have enriched my life through their presence; I hope I have brought just as much to them.

I am very grateful to our staff, Erica Lewis and Karen Williams, for your love and care for our office and all our patients. You make our practice a special place with your beautiful smiles and all that comes with them.

I thank all my patients for your trust and sharing your health journey with me.

Lots of love and thanks to Riley Ali for taking the photograph for the cover. I appreciate your artistic skills and sense. Also thank you Riley for creating the polyphenol tree.

A huge hug and appreciation for Terry Nozick for being my editor. Your help, your time and the wonderful woman you are will always be appreciated.

PREFACE

We are all in this together. We hear this frequently, and it does even apply to your health. Studies show that if your spouse, family, and/or friends are overweight you have a higher risk of becoming overweight yourself. (You can substitute the word "unhealthy" for "overweight" because if someone is overweight, they are unhealthy.) What can you do about this? Make changes. Encourage your spouse, family, and friends to make changes along with you. It will make you, and them, better. It will enhance your quality of life and most likely extend your life, and it will do the same for the people you love.

This book is not meant to be a treatise on weight. Health is a manifestation of a person's lifestyle and there are several variables that dictate whether a person is healthy or not. But the weight of Americans is a visible fact that coincides with the health status of Americans. And it does matter because with increased weight comes increased risk for heart disease, type 2 diabetes, cancers, autoimmune problems, increased risk of non-communicable and even communicable diseases and increased risk of all- cause mortality. This is the result of the microbiome, which you will learn plenty about in this book.

Now is that time for deliberate change, for yourself, your family, and the friends you love. This is the book that will give you the reasons, the scientific studies, and the way to make these deliberate changes. This is not another get-healthy-pep-talk-change-your-diet book. We are living in exciting times, with much research being done on how your diet affects your body. You will read about that in this book. Science has opened our eyes, and we can now see that tiny creatures (microbes) are inside our bodies turning all the cogs!

You can choose health!

Important Points

❖ It is important for you to know why you prefer the taste of the foods that you choose to eat. Taste is of course individual, but each of us trains ourselves to like certain tastes. This is important to keep in mind when you begin eating the different foods that are presented in this book, if they are different from your norm. Allow yourself at least 30 days for your taste buds to get used to eating foods that are natural and seasoned naturally. These foods are not super-saturated with fat, sugar, and salt. If you have become accustomed to eating processed and fast food, then your taste buds are used to getting a large amount of fat, sugar, and salt. (The amount of fat, sugar, and salt in processed and fast foods means that your taste buds have been assaulted over time.) If you consistently eat vegan foods, and no processed or fast foods for 30 straight days, over the course of those days, one day at a time, your taste buds will continue to adjust to how real foods taste. You may even wonder how you could

1

have eaten the processed foods with all the chemicals and super-saturated "flavorings."

❖ "Hyperpalatable" is a term used in the processed food industry for food that contains the right combination of fat, sugar, salt, and carbohydrates that make it a food that people will eat repeatedly, even if they are not hungry. For decades, food scientists have altered the proportions of fats, sugar, salt and carbohydrates to create varied combinations of these four categories to create foods that people actually crave. Hyperpalatable foods are the most desirable foods because they set off the reward centers in your brain, promoting cascades of serotonin and dopamine. Hyperpalatable foods create cravings for that food just like drug addicts have cravings for their drug of choice – it is the same reward/pleasure receptors that get stimulated.

Another way of stating this is, hyperpalatable foods are highly addictive and people will eat them again and again. Hyperpalatable foods are intentionally created to be addictive. It is not by accident that all the hyperpalatable foods that millions of people eat repeatedly are consumed in large quantities, even when they are no longer hungry. It is also not an accident that all the hyperpalatable foods eaten by millions of people are the foods being eaten in greater proportion than minimally processed whole foods. The multi-million-dollar food companies invest heavily to create these hyperpalatable foods that keep you coming back for more with every grocery shopping trip.

You might find motivation in the fact that the food

industry has manipulated your brain, has manipulated you. In America where we all want to be independent and in charge of ourselves, well... the food industry really has control and is in charge of millions of Americans. Are you one of them? Isn't this a good motivator for you to take a stand and take control of your eating habits? The food industry spends millions of dollars on food chemists to create these hyperpalatable foods because these processed foods cause maximum stimulation to the reward center in your brain. It is precisely this stimulation to your reward center that causes you to seek out that food again and again - even though it is a food that has no nutritional value to your body, and does not help your body in any way at all! But instead, it actually causes harm. Hyperpalatable foods- the processed foods and fast-foods, are the foods that have changed the microbiome for millions of people. These are the foods that have allowed disease causing bacteria and fungi to inhabit the intestinal tract and cause chronic health problems, especially gastrointestinal problems. Think about it, in America how prevalent is irritable bowel syndrome, inflammatory bowel disease, metabolic syndrome, type 2 diabetes? Very prevalent! Everyone knows several people who suffer with each of these conditions.

- ❖ It is important to know the difference between salt and sodium and why it even matters. Salt is actually sodium chloride, a combination of two distinct minerals. Proportionately, salt is 40% sodium and 60% chloride. It is the sodium that is a concern for your health if you consume too much, as it is responsible for the fluid volume in your body, in the cells and in the tissues, which is how it

3

influences your blood pressure. But, our bodies need sodium too, because we need to keep some water in our cells and tissues, just not too much. Therefore, sodium is needed in a range; the current range for healthy adults is 2,300mg/day. This matters because keeping your sodium low will help keep your blood pressure low, which makes a difference to your heart and reduces your chances of having a stroke. Using the recipes in the *Mostly Vegan Cookbook*, due out in 2022, will help reduce your sodium as you will be eating more vegetables.

❖ The Standard American Diet will be referred to as the SAD, it is the cause of billions of people having chronic preventable diseases. But, hey, that's okay since there are medications for all of those diseases right? Yes, there are medications for them, but these medications usually affect the liver, kidneys, digestive tract, and some affect your brain. And usually the negative side-effects from a medication are often the cause for needing yet another medication. This is how the majority of Americans, especially the elderly, end up taking multiple medications. And, many people end up taking multiple medications the rest of their lives.

❖ From 2000-2012 a study was conducted with 157,142 American households tracking their food purchases. The results revealed that Americans purchased 61% highly processed foods, 15.9% moderately processed foods and <25% unprocessed or minimally processed foods.[1] Highly processed foods are foods that had multiple ingredients, were man-made and were unrecognizable as being from a plant or animal source. Moderately processed foods contained food additives though the plant or animal source was still identifiable. Minimally processed foods had bare minimum alterations, such as bagged vegetables, eggs, and frozen meats. The study authors noted that the moderately and highly processed foods "were significantly more likely to simultaneously exceed DGA/FDA-recommended limits for saturated fat, sugar, and sodium content compared with purchases of less-processed foods or foods requiring cooking."[2] "DGA/FDA"- Dietary Guidelines for Americans/ Food and Drug Administration.

❖ If you want to make changes to your health you have to make changes to your lifestyle. There are a number of ways to go about bringing these changes into your life. And you do not have to make numerous drastic changes all at once. This point will be expanded on in the chapter "Why Transition People?"

❖ Once you start changing how you are eating, you will realize it is not as hard as you may have anticipated. You'll see you are capable of making changes and eating healthy foods, and that food does not rule you; you have the control to decide what you want to eat.

❖ If you are having a meal that contains animal protein, make the vegetables the main course by going proportionally heavier in vegetables.

❖ The human body is amazing and responds positively when healthy habits replace unhealthy habits. For yourself, your family, and the people you love, you can change your futures, so your lives do not result in endpoints such as the following, which are comparative risk assessment data from the 1999-2002 and 2009-2012 surveys by the National Health And Nutrition Examination Surveys (NHANES) showing "estimated associations of diet and disease from meta-analyses of prospective studies and clinical trials"[3] The survey states, "In 2012, 702,308 cardiometabolic deaths occurred in US adults, including 506,100 from heart disease (371,266 coronary heart disease, 35,019 hypertensive heart disease, and 99.815 other cardiovascular disease), 128,□294 from stroke (16,125 ischemic, 32,591 hemorrhagic, and 79,578 other), and 67,914 from type 2 diabetes".[4]

What Is the Goal of This Book?

My goal is to introduce people to the vegan lifestyle by gradually having them eat vegan meals.

The ultimate goal is not to make you a vegan for life. That is an option, and if you do decide to become vegan for the rest of your life that's great! The ultimate goal is to get you to eat vegan meals one to two times each day. Even that will improve your health as you would be eating meals that are mostly vegetables, some fruits, and some grains. Eating mostly vegan should help you to lose weight and maintain a healthy weight.

If you do decide to become vegan you will definitely be much healthier for it. The results will manifest in a better quality of life for you and good results on your annual blood work from your doctor's office showing your low cholesterol, low A1C/blood glucose levels, a reduction in C-Reactive Protein, and a reduction in counter- productive antibodies and auto-antibodies for people with autoimmune conditions. Additionally, it is possible to maintain a healthy weight while being vegan, which is important for your quality of life, especially as you mature.

Another prioritized goal of this book is to educate you about the numerous health problems Americans face that are mostly preventable. The information in *Mostly Vegan* was written to teach you how to avoid these health problems; the information in this book is your "why" and motivation; and the information in this book is your solution.

Why Teach People to Be Vegan?

I teach people to be vegan to help them change their lifestyle in order to get healthy.

When you are healthy you enjoy a better quality of life. Numerous studies show that quality of life is dependent on health status. America is a wealthy, successful country, but we spend over $9,000.00 per person on healthcare every year, thousands of dollars more per year than people in every other country. Our healthcare costs have only climbed over the last six decades. Isn't it time to ask why?

I also want to help people avoid the prevalent diseases that are mostly preventable. These current health problems are created by the diet that most Western countries consume - a diet high in animal protein, high in saturated and total fats, high in highly-refined and calorie-dense processed foods, and high in simple sugars. This diet is very low in fiber.

Many people who become vegan are specifically motivated by a health problem or problems. Vegan diets have been successful at reversing metabolic syndrome and type 2 diabetes, lowering elevated cholesterol, reducing elevated triglycerides, reducing high blood pressure, reversing obesity, reducing inflammation, and helping to change cardiovascular problems. Many people choose to become vegan for the rest of their lives following a diagnosis of cancer, whether while undergoing or following cancer treatments, in the hopes of avoiding a cancer reoccurrence.

By having a vegan or mostly vegan lifestyle you can avoid most of the prevalent diseases that are lifestyle related and are, for the most part, preventable. The human body is truly amazing, and I have been in awe of it since I was a teenager. When you can live your life feeling great every day, your life can be so much more enjoyable.

Why Transition People?

Many people are not ready to commit to being fully vegan. *Mostly Vegan* gives you options: You don't have to commit to being 100% vegan in order to have regular vegan meals in your diet, and you do not have to be 100% vegan to reap numerous health benefits from a mostly plant-based diet. Realize there are variables about how to eat vegan. Maybe you can eat one to two vegan meals each day, your health will be much better as a result. Another way to structure being mostly vegan is to choose days each week to eat only vegan, like Monday and Thursday or Tues and Wednesday. It is completely up to you, and your schedule, so figure out which days you can stay vegan that would work into your schedule and all the variables that are in your schedule; taking into account your work days, workouts, and family activities/events. Another option is to be vegan for one week or two weeks at a time, or even every other week each month. A key factor is that the days or weeks you are not being vegan, still keep your vegetable intake high. These changes will make a big difference to your health if you consistently eat vegan over a period of time.

There is no set rule about this. Look at these options and think about how keeping vegan meals in your life would work best. And there you have your perfect solution contributing to your health. I have met many people who are "about 90% vegan" and as a result have better health, maintain their weight, do not have problems with blood glucose/A1c, don't have high cholesterol, don't have high blood pressure, and they get to enjoy feeling great every day. This can be you!

What is important if you want to improve your health is to change what you are presently doing that contributed to causing any health problems you currently have. Most likely you have heard the saying, "If you want different results, you have to do things differently." That applies 100% to your health and your lifestyle. If you want to be healthy, you must take steps to create health. You cannot get healthy from a pill. You cannot get healthy from fast food, fatty foods, processed foods, and sugar. Getting healthy requires consistency over time. It is not a quick fix. It is a process that is worth every minute, every day, and every year you put into it.

Eating Evolves - Personally and Nationally

Just because you eat one way at some point in your life does not mean that is the way you will eat the rest of your life. Just think about it. Most likely, you ate a certain way growing up, and at different times in your life you were eating different types of foods. I point this out so that you realize that you are very capable of making changes to the way you eat. This book is filled with facts that I hope will allow you to see why it is absolutely necessary to eat a diet that has more vegetables than any other foods.

I started thinking about my food choices when I was 14, and became a vegetarian for a few years. I hadn't studied nutrition at that point, but I was always trying to make what I thought were healthy food choices. I continued to make healthy choices as I went through acupuncture college, and I still do. Eating healthfully has been a constant factor in my life since age 14. About 20 years ago I had a paleo diet for several years, and then several years later I became vegan for a while. As much as I loved being vegan for several reasons, at a point, I had to re-introduce animal proteins. I have always been either anemic or border-line anemic, and for my body, prolonged periods without vitamin B12 negatively impacts my health. Now, I have days at a time when I am vegan or paleo.

My journey as an Acupuncturist and Herbalist has taught me much along the way. Wanting to always learn more about the human body was definitely a driving factor in choosing this field of holistic health. Throughout my life I have been in awe of the human body and have always desired to understand everything I could about it and be able to take the best possible care of it.

I explain a lot of things to my patients; I want my patients to understand what is happening inside their bodies and how we are going to bring about changes. A priority in my practice is to educate my patients about their diet, as diet always plays a role in chronic health conditions. Your lifestyle and your diet make up your body's environment, internal and external, this is your "microbiome" (more on this later). Each person's microbiome either allows or does not allow diseased states to develop and progress.

Eating is a primal fact of our lives: if you don't eat, you won't survive. Millions of years ago, there weren't a multitude of choices about what to eat. People ate whatever they were able to hunt and whatever edible plants they came upon. People were nomadic out of necessity and moved on when food and water were no longer available. It was a matter of survival. Whatever food they could get their hands on is what they ate, period.

About 12,000 years ago humans started farming. This was the beginning of the Agricultural Age, and it changed human life in many ways. People were able to settle in one location for the first time, allowing food to be produced to meet demand for the first time. This resulted in human population growth. People still had to work hard to get food, but it did not require *as* much physical work nor did it have as high a possibility of failure. For the first time in the existence of human life, the possibility of being able to consistently get calories became a reality.

Food production continued to evolve and people were finally able to consume calories on a consistent basis. And here we are, in the industrialized world, where most of us eat three meals a day, and even snack between these meals. Most people are not starving. In the United States we have the opposite problem: many people are consuming too many calories, which is one of the factors that has led to our current health problems.

In the United States, our current health problems are the culmination of events and fact in human existence that have created the perfect storm to be unhealthy. 1) It is easy to get food. 2) Many of the manufactured foods provide an abundance of calories. 3) Many of the foods have artificial ingredients that cause problems for our organs, and therefore negatively impact our overall health. 4) Sugar consumption has risen dramatically and steadily over the last six decades. This has lead to weight gain and a steady increase in causing and contributing to a number of diseases.
5) Technological developments and modern conveniences have led to us moving our bodies less.

And that is the perfect storm for the health crisis in

America!

The President's Council on Fitness, Sports & Nutrition reported that in all major food categories there was an increase in food production from 1970 to 2008. And in those years the average daily calories per person increased approximately 600 calories. This is important because 600 extra calories every day means 600 calories that get put into storage, which becomes fat, in the body if they are not needed by the body the day they are consumed.

Another very important fact is that since the 1970s, the number of fast-food restaurants has more than doubled. The majority of meals from fast-food restaurants provide an abundance of calories in just one meal. It is recommended that most adult women keep their calories between 1,600-2,400 per day, and adult men consume between 2,000-3,000 calories per day, with the higher end being for people engaged in physical activity. A typical fast-food hamburger meal can be 1,680-1,844 calories and comprising anywhere from 74-103 grams of fat. This is almost all the calories recommended for the day in just one meal!

Obesity Rates - Why We Have to Take a Look

As stated in the beginning of this book, this is not meant to be a treatise on weight and obesity. However, as this book is about health, we have to discuss weight gain and obesity in the United States because the consistent escalation of weight/obesity-same issue, is directly tied to the common and consistent escalation of health problems of Americans. And these way too-common health problems are preventable. Please do not perceive this statement as "picking on" anyone who is overweight or obese. I sincerely love when people have done my *Full Body 30 Day Vegan Cleanse* and lost weight! This information is presented with facts only, no judgment of any kind, and with the intention of helping.

The latest update (up to 2018) from the National Health and Nutrition Survey/NHANES saw only increases in overweight and obese Americans of all age groups, including children, adolescents, young adults, middle-aged adults, and senior citizens.[5] If this was the very first time this trend was seen, it wouldn't be alarming, but it is not new, and it is a situation that has only been escalating for the last 80 years. (To be more factual, humans have steadily gained weight for 12,000 years, as shown in the chapter "Eating Evolves - Personally and Nationally.") Because this is not a new trend it should be alarming that still, in 2021, we are still seeing increases. This data from the latest NHANES shows that "From 1999–2000 through 2017–2018, the age-adjusted prevalence of obesity increased from 30.5% to 42.4%, and the prevalence of severe obesity increased from 4.7% to 9.2%."[6] "The age-adjusted prevalence of obesity was 42.4%, and the age-adjusted prevalence of severe obesity was 9.2% among adults aged 20 and over in the United States in 2017–2018."[7] "Adults aged 40–59 had the highest prevalence of severe obesity."[8] "From 1999–2000 through 2017–2018, the prevalence of both obesity and severe obesity increased among adults."[9] "From 1999–2000 through 2015–2016, a significantly increasing trend in obesity was observed."[10] "The prevalence was 40.0% among younger adults aged 20–39, 44.8% among middle-aged adults aged 40–59, and 42.8% among older adults aged 60 and over."[11]

Since Americans have only increasingly become more overweight and obesity has risen too, this affects the next few generations. Currently, teenagers who live in communities that have high numbers of overweight and obese adults perceive these conditions as "normal." This is understandable if that is what you grow up seeing around you. Their own body perception and what they deem a "healthy" weight and body shape are completely dependent upon the adults they see in their daily life. This is the same perception parents have of their kids; parents who are overweight or obese do not perceive their kids as being overweight or obese, even if they actually are, since it is normal to them. The problem will only continue into generations unless there are deliberate changes in eating and lifestyle factors.

In the same vein, this perception teenagers have is also the perception adults have. As Americans have consistently increased their weight, fewer Americans want to lose weight. This makes sense if you observe that the majority of the people have a larger body size, it becomes acceptable for you to also have a larger body size. This fact is noted in the data from Gallup's Health and Healthcare survey, from November 2019.[12]

In 1952, the American government started trying to help Americans battle weight gain by incorporating steps to inform and bring about changes. The American Heart Association informed Americans that obesity was a "cardiac risk factor modifiable through diet and exercise."[13] In 1974 a doctor wrote an editorial in the *Lancet* journal as a reaction to seeing the increasing weight of Americans. He wrote that in the last 25 years the rates of obesity for adults, adolescents, and children increased "sharply."[14] He further cited that the deleterious effects of obesity increase chronic disease risk, increase morbidity, and increase mortality.[15] He cited sources in writing that obesity comes with high medical costs, as well as social and psychological costs.[16] Also noted was that obesity can persist from childhood into adulthood and is best prevented "starting as early in life as possible."[17]

In 1980 a 10-year plan was initiated by the U.S. Department of Health and Human Services,[18] but did not result in its goals for Americans to lose weight and/or maintain a healthy weight. Ironically, the opposite occurred – Americans gained even more weight. A second 10-year plan was initiated in 1990, also by the U.S. Department of Health and Human Services,[19] with the same results. The American government has been informing Americans for 70 years about the numerous ways obesity has altered health, the quality of life, the costs, and the mortality that go hand-in-hand with obesity. Which leads us to where we are currently.

U.S Statistics show that obese adults made up less than 15% of the U.S. population in 1990. Obesity rates in most states grew to 25% or more by 2010. In 2017, 40% of the U.S. adult population was obese; while the obesity rates in kids and teens grew to 17%. This is important because with excess weight and obesity come disease processes. And while the focus of this book, as well as *Full Body 30 Day Vegan Cleanse*, is not weight loss, the focus is on getting you healthy, and weight loss happens as a result of eating foods as described in this book. The International Agency for Research on Cancer has concluded that being overweight or obese increases the risk for 13 different types of cancers.[20]

The November 2019 Gallup survey discovered that in the previous decade, from 2010-2019, there had been an increase in Americans reporting that they weigh 200 pounds or more.[21] The rate was 28%, up from 24% reported in 2001-2009.[22] To give a little perspective, in 1960-1962, only 0.9% of people were "extremely obese."[23]

In 2016 a review of several studies found that obesity is now causing more premature preventable deaths in the U.S. than smoking.[24] Currently, obesity is known to cause one in five deaths in the United States every year.

In the chapter "Research Links Western Diet to Health Problems" you will read that obesity is now viewed as an autoimmune disorder.

My hope in providing these facts is that this information will help you realize you can make changes for yourself and the people you love to reverse this trend, which has only been moving in one direction for over 70 years. Each person can make these changes and support other people to do the same. This is a very crucial time for the health of Americans and future generations.

Your Microbiome: What It Is, What Influences It, and Why It Matters

The human microbiome is your body's environment – the inside and the outside. Your body's environment is what keeps you healthy … or what allows diseases to occur. Every day you make choices that affect your microbiome.

Your body's environment consists of the bacteria, fungi, viruses, protists and archaea that live in and on your body. Bacteria, fungi, and viruses are organisms you have heard of. Protists are eukaryotic organisms that are not plant, animal or fungus. While archaea are distinct from bacteria due to distinct molecular characteristics, they are also single-celled prokaryotic organisms. There are distinct microbiomes for your skin, lungs, body fluids, mammary glands, ovaries, mouth, and your digestive tract - these distinctive environments are called microbiota. In each of these distinct human microbiotas, there is supposed to be health-promoting organisms, bacteria, fungi, viruses, protists, and archaea. But if the health-promoting organisms are outnumbered by unhealthy strains of bacteria, fungi, viruses, protists, and archaea, inflammation ensues. Inflamed tissues are an altered microbiome, which then is an easier environment for unhealthy organisms to thrive in. The longer the environment is inflamed and houses opportunistic pathogenic organisms, the more the environment gets altered, making it progressively easier for unhealthy strains of organisms to thrive, which leads to disease. Think of it as a perfect storm, with the merging environments acting as catalysts to each other. The chronicity of an inflamed altered microbiota allows the progression to an unhealthy microbiome, leading to over-expression of genes for diseases. A group of scientists, researchers and doctors put it this way: "We now realise that the human microbiota is an overlooked system that makes a significant contribution to human biology and development."[25]

Another group of researchers sequenced bacterial RNA genes from the gut microbiotas of several mammalian species and humans. Their research showed there is evidence that our gut microbiota and its organisms have co-evolved and through that process we require this microbiota to be alive.[26] Another one of their discoveries: "We found that microbiota adaptation to diet is reproducible across different mammalian lineages."[27] This showed that mammals in the same species eating the same diet had the same organisms present in their gut microbiota; likewise, humans eating diets similar to each other also exhibited the same dominant organisms in their gut microbiota. In their concluding statements these researchers wrote, "These results teach us that even fecal samples from mammals living in zoos and human samples from a single self-selected population can provide insights into the factors driving the evolution of the gut microbiome."[28] This all shows the adaptability of the microbiota and its significance to our very existence.

What affects your microbiome? The answer is, everything. The foods you eat, the liquids you drink, alcohol, medications, products used on your skin, and even the air you breathe have an effect. Seems overwhelming, right? But, that is the reality; and that is what it means to be a product of nature, just as every plant is affected by the soil, water, and sunlight that either propel its growth and development or hinder it. Likewise, every animal is affected by the food it eats, the water it drinks, the physical environment it lives in. But compared to plants and animals, humans have many more variables in our daily lives, so there are many more variables that influence our body, brain, and microbiome. The human body is very complex and we still do not have a full understanding about the majority of how our body functions.

Another way to understand the microbiome is how I describe it to my patients, it is all about who has the real estate. Take for example your large intestines it is a tube that runs from the end of the small intestines to the rectum. This organ/tube needs to be thriving with health-promoting bacteria, fungi, viruses, etc., and when these types of microbes live in your intestinal tract, the unhealthy disease-causing organisms do not take up residence. It is all about the real estate and who has it, the good guys or the bad guys? Our intestines/gut microbiota, as well as our whole body/microbiome, are all about the organisms living in and on them. If there is a mass shift in the communities of organisms and those organisms are disease-causing organisms, the gut microbiota - and the whole microbiome consequentially -

will be negatively affected. There is much more information later in this book regarding the intestinal microbiota.

In order to thrive, the human body needs to be in a state of mutualism in which the host and the millions of organisms inhabiting it support each other in a mutually thriving environment. That is what health is.

How Do I Get Calcium?

The recommended daily allowance, or RDA, for calcium set by the Food and Nutrition Board of the Institute of Medicine is up to 1,000 milligrams for adults age 19-50 years, and 1,200 milligrams for people over age 50. Any calcium above this amount does not get utilized or improve bone health. In some other countries the people take in only about 400 milligrams and do not have the levels of osteoporosis we have in America. It is very possible to get the calcium you need from foods other than dairy products. Thanks to marketing, when people think about how much calcium they need, they consider dairy products as the way to get it. But, there is a very good dose of calcium in deep green vegetables. To compare: one cup of cooked kale provides 94 milligrams of calcium; one cup of cooked collard greens has 266 milligrams; while one cup of milk has 300 milligrams. (This is just a very brief example note that all the deep green vegetables provide calcium.)

A very important point to keep in mind is, even though the US is ranked as having the 16th highest dairy consumption out of 100 countries, we are number 1 in rates of osteoporosis. This is because cow's milk has a high phosphorous content, which sets off a cascade of events that result in calcium being drawn out of bone to buffer the toxic levels of phosphate. The World Health Organization and the Food and Agricultural Organization of the United Nations call this the "calcium paradox."[29] For decades it just didn't make sense that the countries with the highest calcium intake had the highest rates of osteoporosis, but once you realize those high levels of phosphate pull calcium out of the bone, it makes sense. North America is also number 1 in osteoporotic hip fractures.[30] As stated in the previous paragraph, 1 cup of milk has 300 milligrams of calcium but, because of the phosphorous in it, your body will not have those 300 milligrams as usable calcium, so you actually net less than that.

Decades of research on bone health and fracture risk have shown that there is more involved than just the bone density. Other contributing factors to bone health are the strength of the bone; the micro-architecture; and a person's muscle mass, fat composition, and diet. A prospective study in the Nurses' Health Study observed that increased oxidative stress was a good indicator of hip fracture.[31] There is also a study that states, "Global indicators of health, education and socioeconomic status are positively correlated with fracture rates suggesting that lifestyles in developed countries might contribute to hip fracture."[32] It makes sense that life in industrialized countries predisposes us to higher rates of osteoporosis as we have hours of inactivity due to modern conveniences, as opposed to the necessary daily physical activity in non-industrialized countries. This gives us a lot to think about.

Just as with bone density is not the only determinant in osteoporosis development, calcium is not the only mineral that factors in. Another group of people with high calcium consumption and a very high incidence of osteoporosis are Eskimos. While they consume a diet very high in calcium via the fish bones they eat on a regular basis, they still have a very high rate of osteoporosis. What Eskimos lack, unless they take in supplements, is the needed amount of Vitamin D.

Current research implicates the importance of Vitamin D intake for healthy bones. When possible, you should spend a short amount of time in the sun to get the Vitamin D you need. We've known for years how vital Vitamin D is for several functions in the body, one of those vital functions is the availability of Vitamin D stores which are necessary for the intestines to be able to absorb the calcium you take in. The usual recommendation for sun time is 15-30 minutes, at mid-day for the best exposure, with about one-third of your skin exposed. If this is not an option, a serving of fish can give you 200-500 IUs of Vitamin D. If you are taking Vitamin D supplements, the current recommendation is for at least 600 IUs (15 mcg) daily. In 2009 there were some medical professionals recommending a higher intake, 2,000 IUs of Vitamin D daily, but more current studies have proven there is not a significant health improvement from such a high dose.

Another very important contributing factor to bone health is Vitamin K, and the best source for it is green leafy vegetables, including kale, Swiss chard, collard greens, dandelion greens, beet tops, spinach, broccoli, parsley, lettuce, and asparagus. In the Nurses' Health Study it was observed that the women who got a minimum of 110 micrograms of Vitamin K every day had a 30% reduced risk of having a bone fracture.[33] One more important fact, Vitamin K2 has been shown to maintain bone strength.[34] The daily recommendation is 120 micrograms.

Other nutrients are vital for healthy bone besides those listed. They play roles in structure and function, and some are necessary catalysts in bone formation. These include magnesium, vitamin C, folate, and potassium, all of which are found in vegetables.

There is currently no consensus on the correct amount of calcium intake to avoid getting osteoporosis. Studies have shown that people with a high dairy intake still get osteoporosis. Other studies compare countries with a very low intake of dairy against countries with a higher dairy intake, and it has been shown that people with a lower or no dairy consumption have a lower rate of osteoporosis. But, to give full disclosure, there are scientific research studies on dairy intake that support both sides. This fact lets us know that your bone health does not come down to just calcium, or consuming dairy products. The truth is that there are many variables that confound the end result of osteoporosis. Some studies are very short term, some are dietary recall, that is, people report their diet after the fact, relying on their memories which are fallible; some studies are on young people in their twenties and look at their dairy intake; some studies are looking at older people and how much dairy they consume at this time in their life while their calcium intake at earlier points in their life is not taken into consideration; some studies have focused on just the calcium intake during the teen years to see if early consumption plays a role in boosting bone health for later years; and across the board it is very difficult to know how much calcium individuals consumed on a daily basis from the time they were teenagers until their sixties. Physical activity is another vital factor for bone health, and most studies on dietary habits do not factor it in.

There are also very good studies on Seventh Day Adventists that look at several different health markers. One such study revealed the results from 25 years of dietary habits and bone health. The conclusion was that the women who were vegan and vegetarian over the 25-year study period did not have an increased risk for wrist fracture (WF) as long as they ate protein-rich foods, nuts, beans, and vegetarian meat analogues.[35] The researchers also concluded that having "a vegetarian diet or diet relatively low in meat consumption does not appear to increase the risk of WF relative to the general population and it may in fact lower the risk of fracture relative to the general population, so long as the diet is high in protein."[36] A good point to keep in mind regarding vegetarians and vegans: as long as they are eating several servings of vegetables and fruits each day, all the anti-oxidants consumed help reduce the oxidative stress and inflammation in the body, which contributes to a lower risk for osteoporosis.

There have been several studies on the effects of soy on bone health. Soy contains isoflavones, which are phytoestrogenic, or plants with estrogen-like effects, though weaker than the estrogen your body makes and hormone replacement therapy. Although there are inconsistencies among studies and results vary with regards to soy being helpful for bone health, there are more studies showing helpful effects from eating soy versus the contrary. Soy isoflavones, or SIs "have demonstrated their viable potential in decreasing bone resorption and enhancing formation. Studies using SI to preserve bone loss show more initial promise under *in vitro* and *in vivo* studies."[37] Whether you are vegan or vegetarian, having some soy in your diet can be helpful.

Overall health plays a crucial role in bone health. It is known that several diseases affect bone health secondarily. Diseases of the gastrointestinal tract such as inflammatory bowel disease, Celiac disease, and anorexia can cause secondary osteoporosis. Endocrine/hormonal disorders like hyperthyroidism, hyperparathyroidism, hypergonadism, cortisol imbalance, growth hormone deficiency or excess as in acromegaly, and diabetes can contribute to development of osteoporosis. Autoimmune diseases such as rheumatoid arthritis, psoriatic arthritis, systemic lupus erythematosus, ankylosing spondylitis, and multiple sclerosis impact bone health and contribute to development of osteoporosis. Liver diseases that affect your bone health are hemachromatosis and chronic liver disease. Kidney disorders that create unhealthy bones are idiopathic hypercalciuria, renal tubular acidosis, and chronic kidney disease.

As with most things in the human body, it really is not as simple as just the dairy or even calcium a person consumes. Physical activity plays a very vital role. Weight-bearing exercises and weight training place a load on the bone, thereby having a positive effect on bone-remodeling and stimulating bone density, bone architecture, and bone mineral content. Soda consumption has a negative effect on bones, usually due to the phosphoric acid they contain, (phosphorous was discussed in the second paragraph in this section). Phosphoric acid is also present in processed foods. Cigarette smoking has a very deleterious effect on bone health. The amount of protein a person eats over the course of years matters. Some medications can alter the bone turn-over rate, decreasing bone density.

How Do I Get Protein in a Vegan Diet?

For many people, one of their biggest concerns is getting enough protein on a vegan diet. Rest assured, it is possible to get the protein you need from a vegan diet, if you have educated yourself about which foods will give you that protein. Listed below are foods that will allow you to be vegan and get the protein you need. Beyond the protein supplied by these foods, all of them are even more valuable for their many phytonutrients.

Soy is popular among vegetarians and vegans because it provides some of the highest amounts of protein and is versatile and delicious. Soy, aka edamame beans, has about 16 grams of protein per cup. Foods made with soy are still high in protein. Tempeh has about 30 grams of protein in a cup and tofu provides about 40 grams per cup. Soy had been shown to lower cholesterol when incorporated into the diet as the main source of protein along with other foods that have cholesterol-lowering effects, which is all vegetables.[38] The people in a 2002 study reduced their low-density lipoprotein cholesterol by 20-30% by eating a diet high in vegetables, soy protein and viscous fibers (beans and legumes).[39] Soy is also a very good source of calcium and iron.

Several years ago soy became very controversial and was thought to induce breast cancer and have negative thyroid effects. But more current research has proved that to be incorrect, and in fact soy has protective effects for breast health and is even helpful for women going through chemotherapy for breast cancer.[40] There is more information about soy in the chapter "Phytonutrients - What Are They?"

Beans are great sources of protein and of my favorite foods because of their plentiful health benefits. There is a wide variety of beans and keeping a variety of them in your life will be very helpful in maintaining your health. There is variation in the grams of protein supplied by various beans, but following are the values for the most popular beans. Cooked beans, grams of protein per cup: black beans 16 grams; red kidney beans 16 grams; pinto beans 16 grams; split peas 16 grams; lentils 17 grams; garbanzo beans 14 grams; great northern white beans 14 grams; and white kidney beans/cannellini beans 18 grams. This is not a complete list, and other beans have similar protein content.

Nuts are a very good source of protein. Each type of nut varies in the amount of protein offered, following is a breakdown for some of the most popular nuts. Raw or roasted, approximate grams per 1 ounce: almonds 6 grams; cashews 4 grams; brazil nuts almost 4 grams; peanuts, raw 7 grams, dry-roasted almost 7 grams; pistachios 6 grams. This is not a complete list of nuts, and other nuts have similar protein content.

Peas are actually a legume that is high in protein and very versatile. Peas boast 7.9 grams of protein per cup. This is the reason why pea protein powder has become a popular option for vegans. You can have peas alone as a snack, or add peas into a rice, pasta, or quinoa dish, stir-fry them and even add them to salads.

Quinoa is one of the only grains with a high protein content, 8 grams per cup. And as with the other protein sources, quinoa is quite versatile. You can eat quinoa with dinner, lunch, and even breakfast. Quinoa can stand alone as a side dish with dinner or lunch, or you can incorporate it into a side dish or even use it as the main dish depending on what you do with it. For breakfast, you can turn it into a hot cereal with some fresh or dried fruit.

Seeds provide protein along with fiber and are a great addition to a vegan lifestyle. Some seeds are perfect for snacking and some can be added into meals, salads, dressings, and smoothies. All seeds contain some protein, and are a good source of healthy fats and fiber. You can't go wrong if you have seeds at least four days a week. Here are the amounts of protein in different seeds per 1 ounce: Sunflower seeds 5 grams; pumpkin seeds 8 grams; sesame seeds 4.8 (almost 5) grams; flax seeds 5 grams; chia seeds 4.7 grams; and hemp seeds 6 grams.

Vegetables also have some protein, though not as much as beans and nuts. You will notice that the vegetables with the highest amounts of protein are the deep green vegetables. Their deep green tones are your clue that these vegetables are the ones you should be eating most often as they supply you with needed phytonutrients. The color of vegetables and fruits is representative of the phytonutrients in that specific vegetable or fruit (there is much more information on this in the chapter "The Rainbow of Phytonutrients.") These values are for 1 cup of cooked vegetables: broccoli, a little over 4 grams; spinach 5 grams; kale, a little over 2 grams; mushrooms, over 3 grams; brussels sprouts, almost 4 grams; Swiss chard, a little over 3 grams; and a medium artichoke, just over 4 grams. These are the vegetables with the most protein, the other vegetables supply less. But vegetables give our bodies so many other needed nutrients, phytonutrients and fiber - good reasons to keep your vegetable intake high and varied.

Getting Enough Other Vital Nutrients

A vegan diet has many health advantages over the omnivore diet, but it lacks some vital nutrients that vegans need to ensure they consume. A vegan diet does not supply adequate amounts of Vitamin D; Vitamin B12; Iron; Zinc; DHA and EPA, the omega 3 fatty acids. These can be consumed through plant supplements. If you are going to be vegan for more than six months at a time, it is highly recommended that you take supplements of these vital nutrients to ensure you are giving your body what is required for optimal function. Being deficient in these nutrients may not be quickly apparent in your health or in blood work, but it will show up at a point and cause health problems if you are vegan for a prolonged period of time. Choline is another nutrient that is necessary for every cell in your body and a vegan diet might supply a low amount of it. There's more on choline at the end of this chapter.

I believe most of our nutrients should come from foods, not supplements, but with regards to these nutrients for long-term vegans that is not the case. There are decades of research revealing how our bodies use and need these nutrients, and this should not be ignored. There is also years' worth of results from people with health problems that could have been avoided if they had healthy levels of these nutrients. Following are the few nutrients you should supplement if you decide to become vegan for more than six months.

Vitamin D is necessary, and studies have shown that many vegans, and vegetarians, are low in Vitamin D. (Though in fairness, even most omnivores are low in Vitamin D.) There is evidence showing how important Vitamin D is in cancer and osteoporosis prevention, and in maintaining a healthy immune system. If you decide to become a vegan, you should ensure you are getting enough Vitamin D either via sunlight or supplement. People who are not vegan get their Vitamin D from seafood, eggs, pork, and fortified yogurt, foods that are not eaten by vegans. As a vegan your best sources of Vitamin D are mushrooms, fortified soy milk, fortified tofu, plant-derived supplements, and 10-15 minutes of sun exposure.

Vitamin B12 is not in many plant foods. Vegetarians and, even more so vegans, are often low in Vitamin B12, which usually manifests later in the form of health problems for prolonged veganism. Vitamin B12 is very important in several physiological processes and is used by every cell in your body. Vitamin B12 plays a crucial role for your central nervous system in making some neurotransmitters. Vitamin B12 is necessary for the production of myelin sheath formation. Myelin sheath is the protective insulator for your brain and spinal cord. Neuropathies, or intense pains, occur when the myelin sheath is inadequate. Vitamin B12 is also required in making red blood cells. A lack of it can cause anemia. Vitamin B12 is needed to regenerate the cells in the intestinal tract, which necessitates a fast cell turnover rate; without healthy renewed cells there is an increased possibility of developing unhealthy bacteria and even fungus, which is usually diagnosed as irritable bowel syndrome or inflammatory bowel disease. For vegans, the best source for taking in your needed Vitamin B12 is through a supplement, and both oral and sublingual have been shown to be effective. A few plant sources of Vitamin B12 are some mushrooms, some algae, and some fermented foods. This is definitely a nutrient that you should supplement, and not take any chances of being deficient in.

Because of the numerous reactions Vitamin B12 is involved in, there are some people who may need to keep some animal protein in their diet, such as those with anemia. Such people need some animal protein to be present to help in production of the red blood cells. People with multiple sclerosis should also consume some animal protein since Vitamin B12 plays a role in the formation of the myelin sheath, although being mostly plant based does help in reducing inflammation that can be very helpful in keeping MS as inactive as possible. One more important note for some people, there are other factors that could be blocking uptake of Vitamin B12, including some medications like proton pump inhibitors, antacids, and H2 blockers.

Iron is not much of a problem for vegans, as was thought by some people in the past. Our bodies absorb iron from animal sources, aka heme iron, more efficiently than from plant sources, or non-heme iron. But, now we know that since vegans eat so many plants that are loaded with vitamin C, all that Vitamin C makes the non-heme iron more bioavailable. Our bodies need iron in order to make the red blood cells that carry oxygen throughout our bodies. Every cell in your body requires oxygen. Every organ requires oxygen. People with anemia don't have enough red blood cells to deliver as much oxygen as the body demands, leaving them feeling tired, unable to concentrate, cold, lightheaded, pale, low energy, and possibly short of breath. Having healthy red blood cells is necessary to live a healthy life. Eating vegan plant-based meals will supply you with a lot of Vitamin C and the iron you need. As a vegan your best sources for iron are as follows: from fruit - tomato sauce not fresh tomatoes; from deep green veggies - Swiss chard, kale, broccoli and collard greens; from dried fruits - apricots, raisins, prunes, and figs; from nuts and seeds - pine nuts, cashews/cashew butter, sunflower seeds, pistachios, chia seeds, hemp seeds, and pumpkin seeds; from legumes - lentils, soybeans, tofu, chickpeas/hummus, and most beans; from grains - quinoa, brown rice, oatmeal, and fortified cereals. And yes, you really can cook some veggies or grains in an iron skillet and increase the iron content of that food.

Zinc is the other mineral we must make sure we are consuming enough of on a vegan diet. Zinc is found and needed in every cell of your body for a multitude of life-sustaining processes. The biggest role zinc plays is being a catalyst for numerous processes - a huge job. Zinc must be consumed daily because there are more than 100 enzymes that require zinc daily in order for them to function. These processes help keep your immune system functioning strongly to avoid infections; are necessary in reproduction for proper development of sperm and eggs; are necessary for the thyroid to make thyroxin hormone, which is responsible for regulating metabolism; are necessary for kids in order to grow; regulates insulin, which is necessary to avoid becoming diabetic; for many women, aids in keeping healthy hair, as low amounts of zinc can cause hair loss; and help create healthy skin.

It's important to know that many of the foods that contain zinc also have phytates in them. The problem with phytates is that they bind to zinc which does not allow our bodies to then absorb the zinc. To ensure you are absorbing as much zinc as your body needs you can eat protein foods that contain zinc to help absorb it. Vegan protein sources that would help are pumpkin seeds, sesame seeds, cashews, almonds, pine nuts and peanuts. Another way to boost your zinc intake as a vegan is to soak certain foods, the soaking releases some of the phytates which then allows better zinc absorption. You can soak your whole grains and beans before cooking them, the over-night soak for the beans accomplishes this. You can also soak nuts and seeds for 1-2 hours before you eat them. You can also eat apples, grapes, and citrus fruits when you eat foods with zinc as they each contain an acid that allows more zinc absorption. The allium vegetables, garlic and onions, also help.

For a vegan diet your best sources of zinc are as follows: nuts and seeds - walnuts, pepitas, peanuts/peanut butter, cashews/cashew butter, almonds/almond butter, pumpkin seeds, and sesame seeds/tahini; from vegetables - green beans, brussels sprouts, spinach, Swiss chard, zucchini, asparagus, broccoli, potatoes, lima beans, and mushrooms; from grains - quinoa and oatmeal; from beans - chick peas/hummus, kidney beans, black beans, white beans, adzuki beans, cannellini beans - all beans contain some zinc. Not to be left out if you are vegan or vegetarian is wheat germ, which is a good source of zinc. You may have noticed that most of these foods high in zinc are also high in iron. These two minerals are often found together.

DHA and **EPA**: DHA or docosahexaenoic acid, and EPA, eicosapentaenoic acid, are healthy fats that your body needs for several functions. Proper brain function requires DHA and EPA for these three jobs: 1) Making neurotransmitters for your brain - the plasma membranes of neurons contain high amounts of DHA as do the terminals for central nervous system signaling. 2) As the basis for some hormones. These fats are necessary for heart health. 3) For their protective anti-inflammatory effects. Studies have shown that vegans have low blood levels of these protective and necessary fats. Most vegans should be supplementing with a microalgae supplement and eating foods that are fortified with DHA. Signs of low levels of these two fats may not manifest for many years, which is why it is far better to proactively supplement with them if you will be vegan for a prolonged period.

Choline may also be a nutrient that should be on the top of the list for anyone who is vegan or vegetarian for a prolonged time. Based on all of my research on nutrients, I believe that given how vital choline is to all your cells and numerous functions in your body it is imperative that you consume the needed amounts. Choline is a necessary element for the cell membrane. It is needed to produce acetylcholine, which is used by every cell in the body and plays a role in so many functions that a whole chapter can get written on just acetylcholine. Briefly, acetylcholine is needed for memory, learning, being alert, executive functions, as well as its role in nerve conduction. As acetylcholine is reliant on choline for its formation you can see how crucial it is to consume proper amounts.

As if that isn't enough, choline is also needed as a methyl donor for the process of methylation. Methylation is a detoxification process which your life depends on. Without methylation, toxins build up in the blood stream, leading to some diseases. There are a number of functions methylation serves and one of those is to reduce homocysteine levels, thereby playing a role in keeping inflammatory signals down. If homocysteine levels are high, inflammation occurs, and this is known to cause arterial damage and increase the risk of cardiovascular disease.

Choline is necessary for the liver too where it serves to remove fats from the liver. But without adequate choline intake, over years, it can lead to a problem called non-alcoholic fatty liver disease, which can lead to cirrhosis. The recommended daily intake for choline is: adult women - 425 mg/day; adult men 550 mg/day; teen girls 400 mg/day, teen boys 550 mg/day; all kids age 9-13 375 mg/day; all kids age 4-8 250mg/day.[41] The majority of foods that supply choline are meat, poultry, fish, eggs, and dairy products, which are all not in the vegan diet. I don't recommend dairy as a way to get choline. Vegans can get choline from soy/tofu, green vegetables, cruciferous vegetables, fruits, potatoes, grains, nuts, seeds, and legumes. Vegetarians can get choline from eggs as well as the sources listed for vegans. Keep in mind though, the amounts of choline in the vegan foods is not as much as the choline from meat, poultry, fish, and eggs.

But supplementing choline is not advised either due to these reasons. First, there are currently inconsistencies among study results over whether choline supplements have been helpful for people suffering with Alzheimer's disease, Parkinson's disease, or other forms of dementia. Second, choline contains trimethylamine, which converts to trimethylamine N-oxide (TMAO), and current research has drawn a relationship between TMAO and the increased risk for cardiovascular disease. Third, and this is related to the second point, supplementation with choline "promoted atherosclerosis"[42] in another study, though the formation of atherosclerosis was dependant on the microbes in the gut (more on that later). The bottom line, based on current research, shows there are other nutrients, minerals, the interaction of the microbe inhabitants, and even other disease processes that all play a part in whether increased choline via supplementation will or will not cause another health problem. But, if you consume the appropriate levels of choline through whole foods it will not cause a problem and at the same time it will safely supply your liver, brain, muscles, and every cell this essential nutrient.

Why This Is Such a Healthy Way to Eat

Eating healthy vegan foods that are plant based will benefit your health dramatically. Eating vegan can lower cholesterol, reduce hypertension, promote weight loss, reduce metabolic syndrome, or change a pre-diabetes status, and be very helpful for a diabetic. A healthy vegan diet can reduce inflammation; reduce your risk for acquiring a chronic disease; reduce your risk of getting an autoimmune disease and reduce autoimmune problems if you already have one or more; and reduce your risk of stroke as you get older. All these listed reasons should be enough for anyone to want to eat more vegetables or maybe be vegan for a short period. There are additional benefits as well.

First, let's start with a plant-based diet. Until September 2019, I had never seen a study showing negative health effects for people eating a diet consisting primarily of plants. In this book, when I refer to "plants" I am referring to mostly vegetables. Fruit is yummy but eating a diet heavy in fruit will not only NOT get you healthy but will cause health problems due to high intake of fructose, the naturally occurring sugar in fruit. People who eat mostly vegetables, grains, beans, and legumes, according to studies, are usually healthier than people who eat the Standard American Diet, or SAD. This study from the University of Oxford, states that among vegans and vegetarians, "We observed lower rates of ischaemic heart disease in fish eaters and vegetarians than in meat eaters, which appears to be at least partly due to lower body mass index and lower rates of high blood pressure, high blood cholesterol, diabetes associated with these diets."[43] these being very good results. But they found a 20% higher risk for stroke among vegetarians and vegans than in meat eaters, which breaks down to three more cases of stroke per 1,000 people over 10 years.[44] But vegans and vegetarians still had all the other very beneficial health markers of lower heart disease while having a decreased risk for heart disease, high blood pressure, decreased risk for increased cholesterol and diabetes. Currently the researchers do not know why there is this slight increased risk for stroke but speculate it could be due to low levels of cholesterol, which does play a very important role in the cell membrane. My take is that it could be other vitamins and minerals that are lower in vegans and vegetarians.

Choline was discussed in the previous chapter, and it was noted that vegans and vegetarians have an increased risk of being deficient in choline. Since it is a necessary catalyst for other biochemical steps, it is possible that the lack of it could have a down-stream effect, years later, on stroke occurrence. Choline is one of the necessary elements of the cell membrane, and if choline is low there will be changes to the functioning of the cell membrane. As you read in the previous chapter, choline is a requirement for the production of acetylcholine, so maybe this is a crucial piece of the puzzle. Or maybe since choline is a needed to keep homocysteine levels down, the higher homocysteine levels could increase the risk for stroke. As is already known, an increased homocysteine level is present with increased inflammation, which causes arterial damage and increases the risk of cardiovascular disease. Arterial damage is a factor in stroke.

At present, this slight increased risk raises more questions. The human body is so intricate and there are many different bio-factors that are required as catalysts to produce or inhibit other bio-factors. As of this date there is not enough research revealing these details.

Second, a plant-based diet that is filled with a large variety of vegetables will provide your body with the numerous phytonutrients it needs to function at its best and be healthy. You should eat a "rainbow of color" of vegetables as the different colors provide a variety of the phytonutrients, and variety is the key to your great health. (More information on phytonutrients can be found in the chapter "Phytonutrients" and more information about the colors of vegetables is in the chapter "The Rainbow of Phytonutrients.")

Third, studies on the microbiome, which you will learn much more about through this book, have concluded that people with the highest intake of vegetables have helpful bacteria in their intestines. People with high vegetable consumption have health-promoting bacteria and don't have the pathogenic, disease-causing bacteria found in people that don't eat as many plants. Also very important, people with the highest vegetable consumption have numerous strains of healthy bacteria in their intestines and more variety of bacteria conveys a broader spectrum of protective and beneficial effects.

Numerous studies compare the gut microbiota of vegans to omnivores, and all have supported the healthy bacteria premise. Two researchers state, "The relationship between diet and the intestinal microbial profile appears to follow a continuum, with vegans displaying a gut microbiota most distinct from that of omnivores, but not always significantly different from that of vegetarians. The vegan gut profile appears to be unique in several characteristics, including a reduced abundance of pathobionts and a greater abundance of protective species."[45] (Pathobionts are bacteria that live in our body, which have the potential to cause disease under certain circumstances.)

Fourth, there are many studies that have proved that eating a vegan diet reduces your risk of several cancers and this is due to a few factors. A) A vegan diet provides a lot of fiber, which lowers colo-rectal cancer risk. B) Since all vegetables provide anti-oxidants, cancer risk is reduced as a result of less reactive oxygen species/free radicals. C) Most vegans eat a lot of vegetables, legumes, beans, fruit, and allium vegetables and all of these have been shown to reduce risk of cancers. Since most vegans are consuming large quantities of these, there is a range of different types of cancers that their diet can protect them from, including mouth, esophagus, lung, stomach, colo-rectal, breast, prostate and kidneys. D) Most vegans maintain a healthy weight and BMI, or body-mass index, this also reduces the risk of cancers. Studies have shown that being over-weight and having a higher BMI increase the chances of getting a cancer.

Fifth, your brain health is directly impacted by the foods you eat. Research studies have shown that reducing bad fats from your diet reduces the risk of developing Alzheimer's disease and even the contrary, that bad fats increases your risk of developing Alzheimer's disease. Combine that with the research showing sugar increases inflammation and think about this double-whammy effect to your brain from unhealthy fats and sugar. Now add in the fact that your body does not easily break down dairy products or processed foods with man-made chemicals, and the result is a cascade of more inflammation. When you put these three factors together it becomes easy to understand how chronic systemic inflammation caused by food has a very large negative effect to your brain. Take a moment and think about any foods that you may eat that are high in fat, high in sugar, and have dairy products in them ... think ice cream, custards, shakes, yogurt. Or look at the foods you eat regularly that are high in bad fats and sugar and are processed with man-made chemicals – the effect will be the same - an irritation to your intestinal tract that causes inflammation in the intestines, and then is a demand on your liver. The result from that is more inflammation and it is known that chronic systemic inflammation plays a role in Alzheimer's disease. The great news is, a number of studies have seen the association between an increase in vegetable intake and reduced risk for developing Alzheimer's disease. (There is more information about the various phytonutrients in vegetables and the many ways those phytonutrients affect the body and cells in the chapter "Phytonutrients – What Are They?" Also, there is more information about Alzheimer's in the chapter "The Gut Microbiota and Your Brain.")

I have never seen a study showing that vegans have

increased risk for hypertension, high cholesterol, cardiovascular disease, and Alzheimer's disease – all diseases that are increased by the SAD. What numerous studies do prove though is a reduced risk for hypertension, reduced cholesterol, reduced cases of cardiovascular disease, reduced A1C/blood glucose markers.[46] [47] Having a lean, mostly plant-based diet, but having some animal protein one to three times per week to provide you with Vitamin B12, is a very healthy way to eat. By eating mostly vegan, your diet will still be mostly whole foods, which have fewer calories and chemicals than processed foods, which is how to lose weight and stay healthy.

While I was writing this book, the *Journal of American Medical Association* published results from a research study proving the benefits of eating a whole-foods diet. The basis for the study was to determine whether people with a genotype pattern or insulin-glucose issue were more successful at losing weight on a healthy low-fat diet or a healthy low-carbohydrate diet. What was fascinating was that everyone lost weight regardless of which approach was taken. The participants ate whole foods, and increased their intake of vegetables and as a result, everyone lost weight. It was a very good study and I think the results are important for every American adult to read because it is not so much one system over another that brought the success, it is that both systems were successful. All you need to do is eat whole foods and especially increase your vegetable intake.[48]

The thousands of scientific research studies that have all reached the same conclusion of overall health from a diet high in vegetable intake are proof that is indisputable. Thousands of studies have shown better heart health, better intestinal health, lower incidence of metabolic problems like metabolic syndrome and type 2 diabetes, lower blood pressure, and more. There are even numerous studies that have resulted in better brain health from a diet high in vegetable consumption. A European study found "regular dietary intake of flavonoid-rich foods and/or beverages has been associated with 50% reduction in the risk of dementia".[49] Another 10-year study on almost 2,000 people that began when they were age 65 or older saw differences between the people who ate higher levels of vegetables and fruits compared with those who had the lowest intake. The people with higher "intake had better cognitive evolution than did subjects in the lowest quartile."[50] Over the 10-year period, the people were examined four times using the same three well-known mental status tests. The conclusions drawn were that the people eating the most flavonoids, constituents only found in plant foods, these people retained better cognition.[51]

How Do You Want to Age?
Your Lifestyle Effects How You Age

There is a vast amount of research proving that our cells, our tissues, and our brain age due to oxidative stress and inflammation which brings about degenerative changes that cause us to age. Your lifestyle is the reason for how your body and brain age. Yes, genes play a role too, and some people are blessed with genes that are hard-wired for longevity. But that is only a small percentage of people. The rest of us are normal in the longevity gene department. And regardless of the longevity gene, the research has proven that people with more oxidative stress and inflammation will experience degenerative changes that will impact their quality of life and how they age.

We all inherit genes from our parents. Within those genes are the predispositions toward certain health problems. These are the health issues that you have seen repeatedly amongst your family members. And since everyone has inherited genes that have a predisposition toward some health disorder, why not just have a healthy lifestyle to prevent whatever your predisposition is?

While you can't do much about the genes you inherit, you can do something about your lifestyle. After 28 years in practice, it is clear to me that how someone takes care of themselves in their 20s reflects in their health in their 40s. What someone does in their 30s reflects into their 50s, and so on ... it really does all matter.

Another very important recent finding is that as our bodies get older, they produce more inflammation. However, this finding appears to be true for people eating the SAD. It is not true for people on a vegan diet. An intervention study that tested levels of inflammatory markers before and after being on a vegan diet showed reductions in all the three inflammatory markers tested after being on a vegan diet.[52] A different study observed that vegans had guts with less pathogenic organisms and more organisms with protective abilities.[53] This study also saw that the vegans had less inflammation, and from that they speculated that the reduced amount of inflammation may have been the determining factor in producing the protective health benefits.[54]

Another recent finding is that too much sitting causes your body to produce more inflammation. Think about how much time you spend sitting each day. Many people sit the entire workday. If you have a long commute to work, factor that in. And what about your weekends, are they activity filled or still more sitting? A sedentary lifestyle will alter your metabolism and cause your body to not utilize the calories you give it – in other words, being sedentary will slow your metabolism down, cause your body to store the calories as fat, (the stored form of calories not needed), and result in weight gain. Excess weight causes inflammation, which changes how your body utilizes insulin, which can lead to more metabolic problems and more inflammation and even more stored fat.

Inflammation causes more oxidation, leading to more free radicals that lead to DNA damage. The more free radicals a person's body has, the more damage to DNA there will be, increasing the chances of developing a cancer. Let's look at this double-edged sword. A person who has a diet with more processed foods will have more inflammation. This inflammation will cause more oxidation and free radicals and increase this person's chances of having cancer. This person that has more free radicals needs as many antioxidants as possible to scavenge the free radicals. But this is usually the type of person that is not eating many vegetables and therefore not getting high amounts of antioxidants. And that is the double-edged sword.

There are several inflammatory makers that are consistently elevated in adults eating the SAD; these same markers are consistently low in vegans. These inflammatory makers are: Interluekin-6, C-reactive protein, TNF-alpha (tumor necrosis factor), TMAO (trimethylamine-N-oxide). Specifically, a vegan diet was associated with decreased plasma TMAO levels.

Let's put just the facts presented in this section together: Sitting causes inflammation, as our body's age they produce more inflammation, more inflammation changes the metabolism and causes more fat storage, increased fat tissue causes – you guessed it – more inflammation, more inflammation and increased fat alter the body's ability to use insulin leading to metabolic syndrome and diabetes. Pretty easy, it's just math, add one factor to the next and the next and the next and it all adds up to the fact that a sedentary life leads to disease. Your diet also plays a role here in reducing the amount of inflammation your body produces as show above in the study comparing vegans to non-vegans.

All of this is very important when you look at the bigger picture- inflammation is the catalyst to all other diseases. Inflammation is the body in an unhealthy state, and this unhealthy microbiome allows other disease processes to develop and thrive.

Also interesting is that the same factors that cause aging – free radicals and inflammation - are the same factors that cause chronic diseases. That is not coincidental but a fact of how your cells are affected by both of those factors.

Foods Affect the Human Microbiome

"Let food by thy medicine and medicine be thy food." This famous quote by Hippocrates is 2,500 years old. In that day, they didn't have the word "microbiome," but Hippocrates clearly saw how foods affect overall health. This is still true today. In fact, even through these 2,500 years and the development of western medicine, it is only now that modern research is reaching the same conclusion that doctors from thousands of years ago reached, that is, your body needs to be treated as a whole. Your body is one organism and the foods you eat will have a direct effect to your entire body - intestines, liver, gall bladder, kidneys, immune system, brain, hormones, and even your bones. That really is the bottom line when it comes to all the research on the microbiome: a healthy lifestyle supports healthy beneficial organisms and an unhealthy lifestyle supports pathogenic organisms that cause disease.

"You are what you eat" is another famous saying. It's true because the foods that we eat are the substrate that bacteria develop from in our large intestines. "Say what?!"

Let's take a look at the digestive process in order to understand this. When you eat, food gets broken down in stages. This begins in your mouth by way of salivary enzymes, then moves on to the stomach, where it is then propelled into the small intestines and with help from liver bile juice and pancreatic enzymes continues to get broken down into a liquid form your cells can use. The final organ to receive the remains of the foods you have eaten is the large intestines. By the time these remnants reach the large intestines, any fiber that has yet to be broken down gets broken down by the bacteria in the large intestines. Their job is to ferment undigested substances that we cannot digest. It is organisms that break down what is left, not cells or tissues from your own body, but organisms. And, this material that is left is what organisms develop from, feed on, and is the catalysts for signaling to the immune system what actions to take. As the gut is the processing plant for the foods you have eaten, it makes sense that it holds the largest inventory of microbes in your body.

The organisms in your gut – mostly bacteria and fungi - break apart the foods you eat to extract the phytonutrients. Though viruses and archaea are also present, future research is needed to provide more information on these organisms as currently the information is mostly on bacteria. Once those phytonutrients have been pulled out, they are in a form cells can use. The organisms that have just worked so hard breaking down the foods you ate also need a fuel supply so they too feed on these phytonutrients. Seems wild, right? But that's how nature is. Think about it, organisms are living things, and all living things have a metabolism and therefore require a fuel source.

There are two givens in this last paragraph. 1) Thousands of years ago the only foods available were natural foods - any organisms in the human body that needed nutrients survived on just natural foods. There were no options. 2) Natural foods -vegetables, fruits, and grains mostly - are the easiest foods for organisms to break down, so it makes sense these would be the sources of nutrition and fuel needed by the organisms that turn all the cogs in our body. Our bodies survived and thrived on natural foods. If our bodies needed processed foods, humans would not have survived.

Just as plant foods have a positive impact on your intestinal microbiota, other types of foods have a negative impact. Vegetables supply phytonutrients that the human body needs and health-promoting organisms need them too. (An upcoming chapter, "Phytonutrients – What Are They?" goes into more detail.) Phytonutrients have powerful antioxidant abilities, which are a constant necessity as our amazing bodies have to deal with free radical scavengers daily.

There are a few types of radical scavengers and each is created in our bodies by a complicated series of steps. Radical scavengers are toxic to our cells, cause chronic inflammation, disease progression, and even lead to cancer. Colon cancer patients displayed higher levels of free radical scavengers and lower levels of antioxidants protecting their body.[55] Another study found that ulcerative colitis patients had increased levels of free radical scavengers in their colon.[56] And there are thousands of other studies concluding the same results: higher amounts of antioxidants protect our bodies against a multitude of diseases.

It's important to know how to protect yourself from free radical scavengers to decrease your odds of getting most diseases and cancers. That protection is eating high amounts of plants. Thousands of research studies have looked into which dietary or chemical substances could interfere with the damage done by radical scavengers, and the conclusion is - plants. Antioxidants from plants do a great job at reducing the amount of radical scavengers thereby reducing the chances of diseases from the damage the radical scavengers cause.[57] [58] [59] [60] [61] [62] [63]

The foods you eat are the material that organisms develop from in your gut microbiota. There is a correlation between having health-promoting organisms and pathogenic-disease-causing organisms and the foods you eat. Your gut microbiota matters because these organisms in your gut determine events affecting your entire body. Health-promoting organisms feed your cells the substances they need, aid in cell-to-cell communication, send signals to dampen inflammatory proteins, and on and on the list goes with cascades of signaling molecules that keep your body functioning at its best. Conversely, pathogenic organisms cause multiple cascades of signaling molecules that have detrimental, disease-producing effects. One such study showed that the gut microbiota of meat-eaters had higher plasma levels of a vascular toxin called trimethylamine-N-oxide (TMAO).[64] The TMAO was produced from the metabolism of L-carnitine, which is plentiful in red meat, by the bacteria in the intestines.[65] These levels of TMAO indicated increased risk of major cardiovascular events and accelerated atherosclerosis in mice.[66] The researchers also gave L-carnitine to people who are vegetarians and saw that their gut microbiota produced significantly less trimethylamine, the precursor to TMAO.[67]

Technology has brought research into a new realm in being able to decipher what the different types of organisms in the gut are as well as their classifications. Researchers now know that the different gut organisms actively take part in their community and actively prevent disease processes or fuel them depending on which specific organism they are. There are three main gut environments/enterotypes; each enterotype is not just one bacterium but is a cluster of several harmonious bacterial species that operate together. The three main enterotypes are: Bacteroides; Prevotella; and Firmicutes. Each of these enterotypes has been repeatedly associated with diet as well as diseases. A gut microbiota "dominated by Bacteroides is adapted to diets high in protein and animal fats".[68] A gut microbiota dominated with Prevotella has adapted to carbohydrate metabolism and vegetarian diets.[69] People with dominance in the Firmicutes are strongly associated with a Western diet[70], and obesity.[71]

Numerous studies have compared the gut microbiota of omnivores to the gut microbiota of vegetarians and vegans. All the studies show differences between the organisms in those distinct microbiota. One of the first studies comparing people on a vegan diet to a Western diet was done in 1987. It was a short-term study that put the participants on either a Western diet, lacto-ovo, or vegan diet for 20 days. By the fourth day the researchers already saw a change in the composition of the organisms in the guts of the participants on the lacto-ovo and vegan diets. By day 20 there was a bigger shift in the microorganisms in the gut toward organisms that are more health promoting in the vegan group.[72] Just 20 days!

There are even some studies comparing the gut

microbiota of vegans to those of vegetarians. And yes, there is a difference in the organisms between these distinct diets. That should be expected since vegans are not consuming any animal protein while vegetarians consume some. What those studies do reveal though is both vegans and vegetarians have lower levels of inflammation and reduced rates of metabolic problems and type 2 diabetes.

Another very important fact is that your gut microbiota, the organisms in your gut, determines what nutrients you absorb from the food you eat. If you eat a diet high in varied plant foods, the gut microbiota will consist of healthy organisms that are capable of absorbing the nutrients from what you eat. Contrasted to a person who has a diet consisting of fast foods, processed foods, fatty foods and sugar, the microbiota created will not contain healthy organisms nor will this microbiota be able to extract nutrients the body needs to function optimally. Built right into this is the reality that the more plant foods eaten, the more plentiful the healthful bacteria becomes, and these healthful bacteria are more efficient at extracting the nutrients from the foods resulting in more nutrients available for you ... one drives the other. Think of it as paying it forward. By eating vegetables, fruits, and grains - foods that are good for you - you have paid it forward to building a healthy environment in your body. As another example of how different types of bacteria end up manifesting processes in our body, the differences in the organisms in the gut microbiota are a key factor in the differences among people in metabolizing drugs, how effective those drugs can be, and even how toxic a drug is from person to person.
The differences in gut microbiotas between omnivores and vegans are fascinating. We read above about the

study discovering the link between the gut microbiota and the development of TMAO leading to increased risk for cardiovascular problems and atherosclerosis. Another study found that a diet based on animal protein alters the intestinal microbiota in more ways than a plant-based diet does. The result from the diet of animal protein showed "increased levels of fecal bile acids, which increased the abundance of bile-tolerant organisms and decreased those species that metabolize dietary plant polysaccharides."[73] There are a few problems if a person has an increase in bile acids in their feces: 1) bile acids increase the permeability of the mucosa in the intestines; 2) the increased permeability alters the microbiota of the intestines becoming an environment that allows/promotes unhealthy organisms; and 3) increased bile acids in the feces is often seen in patients with diarrhea predominant irritable bowel syndrome, or IBS.

On the other hand, numerous studies clearly see the association of a diet high in vegetable intake and good health. As seen earlier, the diet will determine what types of organisms live in your gut. Diets high in fiber from plants are diets that confer a high level of short-chain fatty acids, or SCFAs. The benefits from SCFAs are many. (More information on SCFAs is in the chapter "What's the Deal with Short-Chain Fatty Acids?) One of the SCFAs is butyrate, and there has been an association between high levels of it and the healthful bacteria F. prausnitzii. F. prausnitzii is a type of Firmicutes and a very important commensal bacterium which needs to be abundant in the intestinal microbiota in order to have a healthy digestive tract. There is a correlation between low or depleted levels of F. prausnitzii and several digestive problems, such as IBS, Crohn's Disease, and ulcerative colitis. Per one study, "A strong positive correlation has been found between *F. prausnitzii* and butyrate production in the gastrointestinal tract, suggesting that this species may be associated with higher fiber intake and reduced risk for cardiovascular disease, colon cancer, diabetes and obesity"[74] While "Numerous experimental studies have shown that IBD is strongly correlated with a decrease of *Faecalibacterium prausnitzii* and an increase of *Escherichia coli.*"[75] This specific family from the Firmicutes enterotype is a helpful bacterium while there are other Firmicutes family members which appear to be pathogenic bacteria and are usually present in higher amounts in people that are obese, and/or have type 2 diabetes. It is exactly this situation that makes us realize that the research on the enterotypes and the specific family members in each enterotype is not going to be just a clear-cut, straight-forward reality. Nature is complex. The research is ongoing and in even five years from now the detailed information on the specific families in each of the enterotypes should be very revealing.

What these point to is how the environment in the gut develops into what it is. It is as clear as the demand placed upon the gut that gets resolved out of necessity - the demand being the consumption of fibrous vegetables; the resolution is the development of organisms capable of utilizing the consumed substances. The people that eat more vegetables and dietary fiber place a demand on their digestive tract to break down those foods that are eaten. Just as with omnivores eating meat places a demand on the digestive tract to break down that animal protein. The demand is met by the digestive tract developing the types of organisms it needs to accomplish what is required.

A group of researchers who compared the differences in

gut organisms between carnivores and herbivores put it like this, "These results suggest carnivorous microbiomes have specialized to degrade proteins as an energy source, while herbivorous communities have specialized to synthesize amino acid building blocks."[76] They saw that the environment causes/creates the organisms required to break down the foods being eaten. From this perspective it makes sense, it is a matter of survival. If a person eats predominately vegetables, the body must be able to utilize the nutrients and calories from the eaten source to keep the body alive. The same mechanisms are in place if a person has a diet high in protein; the digestive tract will develop organisms that are efficient at breaking down the proteins. Now think for a moment about processed foods, or high-calorie foods. In order to function properly the human body has a requirement for a certain amount of calories each day. If foods are eaten that provide more calories than are required, of course those calories get stored. If someone is eating calorie-dense foods on a regular basis, organisms that are efficient at storing calories will dominate due to the demand placed on the gut. These are the types of organisms that have been seen in numerous studies of people who are overweight, their intestines houses organisms that are efficient at storing calories. These organisms do not specialize in utilizing the calories. These would be the people you hear saying, "I put on weight if I even look at a piece of cake." I think we all know people like this. And it does seem unfair. But, know that your ability to alter your microbiota is possible as many scientists and researchers have seen in numerous studies. All it takes is eating foods to change the gut microbiota – which is the point of this book.

There are volumes of research proving that your gut

microbiota becomes what it currently is and gets altered by the foods you eat. While foods are the biggest determinant of the gut microbiota, liquids do contribute to the gut microbiota make-up especially if sugar-filled drinks are regularly consumed or alcohol, or diet drinks. Everything ingested has impact to the gut microbiota. Drugs of all types alter the microbiota too but that is not the focus of this book.

In this section and throughout the book, the scientific research studies cited are only a very small percentage of the studies done that draw similar results. None of these studies was a one-off, all had consistent reproducible results to studies done before and after. All the studies hold important information that should be influencing the changes we should make to our diets if we want to be healthy.

The field of studies looking at the relationships between the organisms and their influence on the entire body is still in its infancy. In 10 more years, what will be learned about the effects of organisms to our bodies from the organisms that live in it will amaze us. Now and in the future, all this information should be used to guide our choices for ourselves and our families.

The Western Diet's Influence on the Microbiome

While the Standard American Diet, or SAD, is *the* cause of our health crisis today, it actually started several decades ago. Even after seeing the results of the SAD for decades and becoming a progressively sicker country, right now in 2021, the U.S has not yet reached the turning point. The same health mistakes are continuing. Americans have steadily increased their consumption of sugar, high fructose corn syrup, alcohol, processed foods, animal protein, and fat while decreasing intake of vegetables, fruits, and whole grains.

A group of researchers combed through epidemiological and scientific studies to be able to see the relationship of risky behaviors and mortality rates. One of the results gleaned was that mortality in the U.S increased from 14% or 300,000 deaths in 1990, to 16% or 400,000 deaths in 2000, and the causative factors for this increase is thought to be poor diet quality and physical inactivity.[77] This same group of researchers concluded: "These analyses show that smoking remains the leading cause of mortality. However, poor diet and physical inactivity may soon overtake tobacco as the leading cause of death. These findings, along with escalating health care costs and aging population, argue persuasively that the need to establish a more preventive orientation in the US health care and public health systems has become more urgent."[78]

A large study on the health of Americans that looked at our health trends over the 30-year period of 1990-2010 was published in 2013. This group of more than 120 doctors and scientists determined that our biggest risk factor for disease, mortality, and disabilities is our diet.[79] This large study came to the conclusion that our SAD is the most dangerous factor to our health.[80] The researchers wrote that the most damaging factors from the SAD are that it is:

* ❖ Low in fruit
* ❖ Low in vegetables
* ❖ Low in nuts and seeds
* ❖ High in processed meats
* ❖ High in sodium
* ❖ High in trans-fats
* ❖ Low in whole grains
* ❖ Low in fiber[81]

And this is from the *Journal of Royal Medicine*: "The number of diverse gut microbial species is diminished in nearly all modern chronic conditions studied." The "Western diet, rich in animal protein, fats and artificial additives, and lacking in fibre, beneficial microbes, plant phytochemicals, vitamins and minerals, is thought to drive these conditions by encouraging gut dysbiosis. Evidence from recent dietary intervention studies suggest adopting a plant-based, minimally processed high-fibre diet may rapidly reverse the effects of meat-based diets on the gut Microbiome."[82] "Dysbiosis" refers to an imbalance in microbes due to a perturbation in the microbial environment away from a symbiotic relationship between the host and microbes to a relationship that is bad and unhealthy.

Here too, when researching scientific studies that look at the relationship of Americans' health and our SAD, there are almost 300 million results. You will continue to read in this book how the SAD is affecting our health, but for now let's move on to a different aspect of the SAD that makes a difference to our health.

Ingredients found in processed foods, emulsifiers specifically, have been shown in several scientific studies to alter the intestinal environment causing inflammation in the intestines of mice. (The studies on emulsifiers are restricted to animals, mice are used most often.) Emulsifiers are widely used in processed foods as a way to get the ingredients to mix well together, create interesting textures and tastes and prolonged shelf life. Interestingly, emulsifiers cannot be digested and eliminated through the feces. It makes sense that emulsifiers cannot get broken down – for this very reason they prolong shelf-life.

Here are conclusions from just a small sampling of these studies. In one study, the researchers wrote, "New studies in murine models suggest that dietary emulsifiers may trigger the gut inflammatory cascade. New studies of restriction diets in patients have shown a relationship between dietary intake, symptoms, and bowel inflammation."[83]
Another study concluded with the similar results. In this

study, mice were given small amounts of two commonly used emulsifiers, and chronic inflammation ensued, which then changed which types of bacteria were living in the intestines of the mice. As a result of these changes, the mice became obese and had metabolic syndrome.[84] The authors concluded, "These results support the emerging concept that perturbed host-microbiota interactions resulting in low-grade inflammation can promote adiposity and its associated metabolic effects. Moreover, they suggest that the broad use of emulsifying agents might be contributing to an increased societal incidence of obesity/metabolic syndrome and other chronic inflammatory diseases."[85]

One of the researchers in the previous study was later involved in another study looking at emulsifiers. At the conclusion of the study he and his colleagues wrote this, emulsifiers "promoted microbiota encroachment and increased levels of pro-inflammatory flagellin and lipopolysaccharide (LPS), which correlated with a change in microbiota composition and intestinal inflammation. Such alterations promoted colitis in mice genetically predisposed to this disorder, and induced low-grade inflammation and metabolic syndrome"[86] Polysorbate-80, a commonly used emulsifier, was seen to alter the pathogenic levels of E. coli by enabling E.coli to increase its concentration, as well as enabled E.coli to increase its ability to translocate across the gut epithelial cells.[87] This increased concentration of E.coli is a dysbiotic state that allows diseases to take place.

It has been noted by several researchers that now that Japan has been eating a more Western diet there are more cases of Crohn's Disease, or CD, there - as has been seen in America and Europe over the last four decades. In 2013, four gastroenterologists at the University of Liverpool wrote, "We suggest that consumption of emulsifiers in processed foods may promote CD by increasing bacterial translocation. This is supported by evidence that geographical variation in CD correlates with emulsifier consumption as does the increasing incidence of CD in Japan"[88]

A more recent study simulating a human intestinal microbiota saw fast changes to the tested microbiota, which was specifically due to the emulsifiers being used in this study. The researchers concluded by stating that the use of the emulsifiers indicated "that the microbiota can be directly impacted by these commonly used food additives, in a manner that subsequently drives intestinal inflammation."[89] Additionally, "Administration of substances that alter microbiota composition, including the synthetic dietary emulsifiers polysorbate 80 (P80) and carboxymethylcellulose (CMC), can promote such inflammatory disorders."

There is no disputing that emulsifiers impact the microbiota of mice; and they have been seen to affect the human microbiota as well, this is information gleaned from epidemiological studies as that is the limit of experimentation on humans with regards to emulsifiers.

There are thousands of studies showing changes to the human microbiome from the Western diet. The above are a few examples of research studies that prove how interrelated our microbiome is with the foods we eat, and how affected our gut is by synthetic products.

Another synthetic additive in many foods is artificial sweeteners. This is important because of their prevalent use in foods consumed through the Western diet. With regards to this synthetic compound there are also many studies that show how non-caloric artificial sweeteners change the gut microbiome.

In one study, where microbes taken from mice fed saccharin were transplanted to germ-free mice, the experimental transplant-recipient mice "developed glucose intolerance and their Microbiomes reflected many of the changes observed in the donors, as compared to those receiving Microbiomes of control mice."[90] These researchers found it interesting that as a direct consequence of the altered microbiota, the experimental transplant mice experienced metabolic syndrome, obesity, and diabetes.[91] This same group of researchers also did some experimenting with people. For people who consumed non-caloric artificial sweeteners, there were consistent alterations in body-mass index, blood pressure, A1C and blood glucose levels, as well as changes in bacterial strains and how much of them.[92] All these results were different for people who did not consume non-caloric artificial sweeteners.[93]

Consistent results have been seen by other research studies as well. A well-known study, the San Antonio Heart Study, proved that the risk of weight gain and even obesity was greater for the people who regularly consumed beverages that were artificially sweetened compared to people who did not.[94] Another group of researchers ran experiments comparing glucose homeostasis in animals given either saccharin or glucose. They found that after consuming saccharin the rats had more of an elevation in their blood glucose levels than the rats given glucose.[95] These researchers think saccharin changes how glucose gets processed and as a result alters glucose homeostasis.[96] Another group of researchers found results consistent with numerous studies and wrote, "Our data are consistent with findings of previous studies that have shown an association between diet soft drink consumption and metabolic syndrome and its components."[97] What all the studies show repeatedly is that artificial sweeteners contribute an increased risk for getting metabolic syndrome, gaining weight, and an increased chance of getting type 2 diabetes. These health situations are linked as a result of biological processes that take place in the body from the artificial sweeteners.

The trillions of microbes in the gut are the result of long-term dietary patterns that have allowed those specific microbes to exist. The gut microbiota and host co-evolve. People with type 2 diabetes carry bacterial strains that people without type 2 diabetes do not have. Obesity is the result of a microbiota that houses pathogenic bacteria also, as you will read about coming up.

The research studies cited here are a very small sampling of the studies that have been done which all concluded with similar results. There has been tremendous interest in the gut microbiota and its influence on the health of the entire body, so much so that between 2013-2017, there were 12,900 published papers on the topic.[98] "In 2017, approximately 4,000 papers focusing on the gut microbiota were published."[99] The largest focus of these studies was on the bacterial aspect.[100]

These studies have crucial information that needs to be implemented into our lives if we are to turn health around for Americans. There is no arguing with the results from thousands of studies proving that the SAD directly damages our health. It's been proven that foods eaten create the microbiota of the gut, which in turn creates the microbiome, which is the environment of the whole body. I also see the direct effect food has on peoples' health in my practice, where I treat people with chronic conditions. Once I put them on herbs and help them to change their diet, their health changes.

Modern Research Reveals

In the last 25 years, several research studies have been able to decipher the different types of bacteria that live within the intestinal tract. These studies show differences across the board in organisms that live in people with digestive problems compared to people who do not have digestive problems. Which makes sense since the environment in the intestines of people with digestive problems will be different and house different types of organisms than people who do not have digestive problems. This is also the reason for fecal transplants. Yes, fecal transplants. This is not a brand new therapy as it was used thousands of years ago in China. It is exactly as it sounds, transplanting feces from people with healthy bacterial species into people with digestive disorders. Fecal transplants are very helpful for people with Clostridium Difficile infection/C.Diff, Crohn's disease, Colitis, and Irritable Bowel Syndrome/IBS. It has a very high success rate, lending proof to the fact that the organisms make up the environment.

I tell my patients that their intestinal tract is like a

compost bin. You start your compost bin by putting natural food scraps into it and then one day when you go to deposit more scraps you see there are some little bugs crawling around. Then a few weeks later you see those bugs and some new ones. And then two months later you notice earth worms. Yet, you never put earth worms into the compost bin. How did they get there? They got there because the environment allowed it. All those natural food scraps have been going through breakdown from bacteria, and eventually worms/parasites. Our intestinal tract works the same way.

Our intestinal tract, the large intestines specifically, is the organ that is the dumpster; it carries the waste products out of our body. So, it makes sense that there will be bacteria there. What matters is the types of bacteria. Since this is the depository for the foods you eat, of course the foods you eat make all the difference to what that waste is. If you eat some broccoli, the bacteria that are capable of breaking it down are different from the bacteria that can break down a steak (as was explained in the section "Foods Affect the Human Microbiome.")
We are fortunate to be living at a time when the scientific research on organisms and the human body is so mind-blowing that it is almost hard to believe. That is the role of science, to always open our eyes to gain an understanding. As hard as it may be to believe some of the mind-blowing reality of organisms and the results garnered by current research realize, it was just as hard in 1676 when Antony Leeuwenhoek discovered bacteria for the first time. His already established professional relationship with the Royal Society of London became dubious as the members did not believe his claim of seeing organisms too small to be seen by the naked eye. Some of this current research may be hard to accept as

real and true, but in 20 years, it will be so easily accepted that it will be common knowledge to all people.

If it is new information to you that the organisms in your gut become those organisms as a result of the foods eaten, then understandably, this is a weird reality to grasp. Hopefully this weird reality will bring about a paradigm shift in how you perceive and then treat your body. It is the reality many research scientists want you to know. These scientists, from different states and even different countries, have repeatedly gotten the same results upon comparing people with different diets and the resultant microbiota. That result is: the diet drives what organisms live in the gut.[101] [102] [103]

Eighteen people in the Calorie Restriction Club participated in a study that compared their gut microbiotas. These people were chosen as they are meticulous about recording the foods they eat and even the weight of those foods thus drawing a clearer line from foods to organisms. Because of the meticulously kept records, the researchers could clearly see how the gut environment was affected by differing amounts of animal proteins or plant foods. The study concluded with the researchers stating, "These results confirm that within a single free-living species, both the structure and function of the gut microbiome are significantly associated with dietary intake."[104]

A chosen topic for many researchers is the comparison of the gut microbiota of omnivores vs. vegans, or for the purpose of a study, putting omnivores on a vegan diet to observe the changes in their gut flora and then comparing these organisms with the organisms from the people who remained omnivores. Here is a study that did just that:

Participants were placed on one of two diets. The animal-based group ate animal products for three meals each day along with snacks from animal products. The plant-based group had cereal for breakfast and then rice, vegetables, and lentils for their lunch and dinner; their snacks were fresh or dried fruit. The participants ate these diets for five consecutive days. In just five days there were changes to the intestinal microbiota in which types of organisms predominated. "The animal-based diet increased the abundance of bile-tolerant microorganisms (Alistipes, Bilophila and Bacteroides) and decreased the levels of Firmicutes that metabolize dietary plant polysaccharides (Roseburia, Eubacterium rectale and Ruminococcus bromii). Microbial activity mirrored differences between herbivorous and carnivorous mammals, reflecting trade-offs between carbohydrate and protein fermentation."[105]

This development in just those five days in the people in the animal-based group developing organisms that were bile-tolerant was a shift in their intestinal microbiota toward an environment that is seen in people with digestive disorders. These researchers concluded there was a "significant" increase in bile acid production;[106] an increase in bile salt hydrolases;[107] and an increase in a secondary metabolite that is "known to promote DNA damage and hepatic carcinomas."[108] The problems seen for people with higher amounts of bile acids, as discussed earlier in the section "Foods Affect the Human Microbiome" are: 1) bile acids increase the permeability of the mucosa in the intestines; 2) the increased permeability alters the microbiota of the intestines, becoming an environment that allows/promotes unhealthy organisms; and 3) increased bile acids in the feces is often seen in patients with diarrhea predominant

Irritable Bowel Syndrome/IBS. One more point made by these researchers was "we found that microbiota changes on the animal-based diet could be linked to altered fecal bile acid profiles and the potential for human enteric disease"[109] (intestinal disease).

Another similar design study switched the diets of African Americans and rural South Africans to see whether the extreme differences in their diets would change the microbial composition of their gut microbiota. These researchers were interested to see if diet was a probable contributing factor in African Americans experiencing a much higher rate of colon cancer than the people of rural South Africa. For two weeks the participants ate the foods the other group was accustomed to eating; the African Americans ate a high-fiber, low-fat African diet and the rural South Africans ate a high-fat, low-fiber "western style" diet. "In comparison with their usual diets, the food changes resulted in remarkable reciprocal changes in mucosal biomarkers of cancer risk and in aspects of the microbiota and metabolome known to affect cancer risk, best illustrated by increased saccharolytic fermentation and butyrogenesis, and suppressed secondary bile acid synthesis in the African Americans."[110]

As seen in the earlier sections, this is just a small amount of the research studies on this topic that all conclude with similar results, that the microbes in the gut are the result of the foods eaten.

Research Links Western Diet to Health Problems

The Standard American Diet, or SAD, has been the cause of digestive disorders for millions of people, as numerous studies have proved that the SAD allows unhealthy, pathogenic organisms to thrive in the intestinal tract.

As Americans continue to experience increasing numbers of chronic health problems, researchers continue to conduct studies that will shed light on why we are experiencing for the first time in our history the very high levels of diseases that are mostly preventable. This is also the first time in history that parents are outliving their kids – this is due to the obesity epidemic and the related chronic health problems that obesity causes.[111] The SAD has been linked to most of the chronic health problems being experienced in record numbers by Americans, and at younger ages too. These studies are proof that foods affect the human microbiome.

Absolutely crucial to a healthy body is the relationship between the gut microbiota and the immune system, which many scientists have seen in their research. When a person's intestinal tract has certain types of organisms or too much of a certain type, or a lack of diversity, the immune system is affected. Have you ever stopped to think how your immune system works? Or why some people have certain diseases? Or why some people have autoimmune problems? Or why some people seem to never get sick and some people are sick often?

Before you read this section, this is the perfect opportunity for you to ask yourself, "If a magic wizard offered me health, would I take it?"

Not only have scientific studies noted the differences in the gut microbiota of omnivores compared to vegetarians, there are also many studies that look at the differences in health issues amongst omnivores compared to vegans, and the results are eye opening. One such study concluded, "This brief lifestyle intervention, including a vegan diet rich in fresh fruits and vegetables, whole grains and various legumes, nuts and seeds, significantly improved health risk factors and reduced systemic inflammation as measured by circulating CRP.[112] "Additionally, those participants who had a vegan diet prior to the intervention had the lowest CRP risk coming into the program."[113] CRP, or C-reactive protein, is an indicator of systemic inflammation. Elevated levels of CRP are seen in a number of health problems, including infections and cancer. It is also an indicator of inflammation in the arteries of the heart, pointing toward possible heart attack if elevated.

We now know that the difference in the types of organisms in a person's gut is completely dependent on the foods being eaten. Just as we now know that those differences in organisms plays a role in disease states. There are many scientific researchers who have made a comment in their published papers that is similar to what these researchers claim, and that is, "Gut dysbiosis, resulting from continued perturbations to the intestinal ecosystem, is implicated in disease states"[114]

Many researchers have come to see that there is a direct relationship between a person's intestinal microbiota and their immune system. This relationship is not a static one but instead is continually evolving under the influence of the foods that are eaten. One group of researchers put it this way: "Compelling evidence obtained over the past 3 years demonstrates that the intestinal microbiota is able to shape the immune system to maintain homeostasis in healthy states or promote inflammation when the composition of the microbial community becomes imbalanced (dysbiosis)"[115]

Another group of researchers reached this conclusion: "The mammalian gut represents a complex ecosystem consisting of an extraordinary number of resident commensal bacteria existing in homeostasis with the host's immune system. Most impressive about this relationship may be the concept that the host not only tolerates, but has evolved to require colonization by beneficial microorganisms, known as commensals, for various aspects of immune development and function. The microbiota provides critical signals that promote maturation of immune cells and tissues, leading to protection from infections by pathogens."[116]

The human body is absolutely fascinating, and the more we learn about it, the more we learn how complex it is. Research on the gut microbiota and its influence on health and disease is a very hot area of research because even though it is in its infancy, the results showing the causal links between the gut and health and the gut and disease are pretty telling and consistent. When it comes to the relationship between the gut microbiota and the immune system one group of researchers wrote, "The microbial community in the mammalian gut is a complex and dynamic system crucial for the development and maturation of both systemic and mucosal immune responses. Therefore, the complex interaction between available nutrients, the microbiota, and the immune system are central regulators in maintaining homeostasis and fighting against invading pathogens at mucosal sites."[117]

Autoimmune diseases have been a growing health problem in America over the past four decades, particularly in western countries, and particularly among women. An autoimmune disease is present when the immune system does not operate in a manner that protects the body but is instead damaging tissues and/or organs. This steady increase in autoimmune problems has been linked to the composition of the gut microbiota which is a consequence of a modern lifestyle causing dysregulation of the immune system.[118] One group of scientists was able to ascertain "significant differences in the abundance of nine bacterial taxa, of which four were found to be different in seropositive versus seronegative cohorts"[119] among people being tested for autoimmune antibodies. While in Japan a group of scientists discovered this when they compared the gut microbiotas of healthy people to those of people with Multiple Sclerosis, "we found 21 species that showed significant differences in relative abundance between the MS20 and HC40 samples. On comparing MS samples to the 158 longitudinal HC18 samples, the differences were found to be reproducibly significant for most of the species."[120] "MS20" is participants with Multiple Sclerosis. "HC40" refers to healthy control-participants without Multiple Sclerosis. Another group of researchers concluded, "The current evidence supports the notion that changes or alterations of the microbial species that form part of the intestinal microbiota will affect the balance of" immune regulatory cells "which could modify the immune response of non-intestinal autoimmune diseases."[121] Their conclusion was that inflammatory cascades cause a non-intestinal autoimmune response. "The major message of this review is that the abundant data support the notion that the intestine is a critical organ for the appropriate immune balance and for the prevention of non-intestinal autoimmune diseases."[122]

There are over 100 different autoimmune diseases. Even now in 2021, it is unknown what "causes" them to occur. Though, now that researchers and scientists have been able to detect differences in the microbes living in people, most diseases are now viewed in a different light; and while the definitive causal links have been proven, western medicine will still not definitively claim what the cause of autoimmune problems are. Several reproducible studies have seen that people with autoimmune diseases have gut microbiotas that have different microbes when compared to the gut microbiota of people that do not have autoimmune problems. This information has allowed a new understanding of autoimmune problems and brought them into a realm in which we can start to figure out solutions for them. A common thread among several different autoimmune diseases is an intestinal environment of dysbiosis that lacks bacterial diversity.[123] Some of the autoimmune diseases that have been linked to this lack of bacterial diversity are inflammatory bowel disease,[124] atopic eczema,[125] type 1 diabetes,[126] type 2 diabetes,[127] psoriatic arthritis, [128] arterial stiffness,[129] and obesity.[130]

Rheumatoid arthritis, or RA, is another of the known autoimmune diseases. It has been recognized since 1800, but the steady rise in incidence is a cause of concern due to its debilitating effects. Modern research traces the association between a dysbiotic microbiota to the increased rate of rheumatoid arthritis. "Changes in the microbiome due to changing lifestyle and dietary habits have led to immunological imbalances. This dysbiosis can influence the immunological damage in conditions like RA and inflammatory bowel disease".[131]

In scientific study after study, this same conclusion has been reached again and again. Another group of researchers wrote, "Altered microbiota composition or dysbiosis is suspected to be implicated in the pathogenesis of chronic inflammatory diseases, such as spondyloarthritis (SpA) and rheumatoid arthritis (RA)."[132] "Our results suggest that distinctive dysbiosis characterise both SpA and RA and evidence a reproducible increase in *R. gnavus* that appears specific for SpA and a marker of disease activity. This observation is consistent with the known proinflammatory role of this bacteria and its association with IBD. It may provide an explanation for the link that exists between SpA and IBD."[133] "IBD"- Inflammatory Bowel Disease.
There exist hundreds more studies reaching that same conclusion regarding the link between RA and the microbes living in the gut microbiota. These studies can be summed up by stating that the intestinal microbes have proven to play a role in the disease process of

rheumatoid arthritis.[134] [135] In 2010, a study was performed using two groups of mice to determine if the gut environment was a determining factor in setting off an inflammatory response that would cause autoimmune arthritis. The researchers stated that for autoimmune arthritis to develop an inflammatory cascade gets put into motion by specific signals from immune cells which "depends critically on gut microbes"[136]

And here is another important fact; people with rheumatoid arthritis have twice the risk for developing cardiovascular problems such as heart attacks, strokes, and atherosclerosis. In addition, the reality in clinical practice and studies too show that people with gout also have a higher rate of rheumatoid arthritis. These are co-morbid factors, diseases that often exist together. When the body is viewed as a whole and not separate parts, the fact that most chronic diseases have co-morbid factors makes perfect sense. Stated another way, your microbiome can be the residence for organisms that promote the health of your organism/microbiome, or your microbiome can be the residence for organisms that promote disease. The microbiome consumed by disease-causing micro-organisms produces changes to organs, glands, and tissues which will then always affect other organs, glands, and tissues – this is why co-morbid factors exist.

Obesity is also being viewed as an autoimmune problem that exists due to the alterations of gut microbes. From my perspective, this is good news since the gut microbes can be altered by the diet! That is exciting! (More about this in later sections.) Adipose tissue, or body fat, is known to be an endocrine organ because it secretes certain hormones. Adipose tissue is also known to be an immune organ because it directs immune system activity.

Now that obesity is viewed as an autoimmune condition, like all autoimmune problems, healthcare professionals know it is multi-factorial. It does come down to the organisms in the gut yes, but those organisms set off a number of events in the body. This was discussed in the previous paragraphs regarding rheumatoid arthritis, but in this scenario the gut microbes create alterations that manifest with an increase in weight. The factors that get disturbed from a homeostatic state to an obese state are changes in how calories get used; immune system dysregulation; inflammatory events; and gut hormonal changes. Let's take a look at some of the conclusions reached regarding the gut microbiota and its role in obesity.

Many scientific studies conclude that there is a reduction in Bacteroidetes in people with obesity compared to lean people, and that once people lose weight there is a shift in the organisms and Bacteroidetes increases.[137] This referenced study was done on mice and people, and then this same group of researchers, when looking at just mice saw, that "through metagenomic and biochemical analyses that these changes affect the metabolic potential of the mouse gut microbiota. Our results indicate that the obese microbiome has an increased capacity to harvest energy from the diet."[138] The Firmicutes group of bacteria proved that they store more of the energy/calories taken in compared to other microbes that live in leaner mice, and people. Then these researchers were able to transplant the gut microbiotas from the obese mice to lean mice and the result was "a significantly greater increase in total body fat than colonization with a 'lean microbiota'. These results identify the gut microbiota as an additional contributing factor to the pathophysiology of obesity."[139] The shift in micro-organisms that has repeatedly been observed in numerous scientific studies is a decrease in the Bacteroidetes group as the Firmicutes group increases in the obese microbiota.

Another common feature seen in the gut microbiota of people who are obese is a lack of diversity of bacteria when compared to the gut microbiota of people who are lean. This fact has been reproduced numerous times by different researchers and scientists.[140] [141] [142] Recall that just a few pages ago you read that a common thread among several different autoimmune diseases is an intestinal environment of dysbiosis that lacks bacterial diversity. A study comparing children in Africa on a traditional African diet with European children on a Western diet revealed, "The nutrient-rich, fiber-poor Western diet reduced the diversity of the gut microbiota, whereas the fiber-rich diet was associated with an increased diversity of the gut microbiota, resulting in a concomitant increase in the diversity of enzymes that can produce a variety of SCFAs (short-chain fatty acids)."[143] Two very important distinctions from this study as it relates to obesity 1) the lack of bacterial diversity from a Western diet, and 2) the ratio of Bacteroidetes to Firmicutes was shifted in these children, with the African children having higher Bacteroidetes:Firmicutes ratio and the reverse ratio in the European children.[144] Recall that Firmicutes are very good at storing calories.

Another factor driven by the gut microbiota is immune system dysregulation due to the body storing too many calories. This seems to take on a life of its own once certain steps have been put in motion. A dysbiotic gut causes the immune system to go into overdrive and produce several biochemicals that end up causing more harm to the body. Without getting too technical, let's take look at some of the biochemicals that become altered due to unhealthy organisms in the gut.

Cells referred to as T-reg/T-regulatory cells, are responsible for control of the immune system, maintaining self-tolerance, and preventing autoimmune problems. T-reg cells are directly affected by pathogenic organisms in the gut. The T-reg cell activity gets decreased in response to dysbiosis, a perturbed gut environment housed by pathogenic bacteria, taking away the regulatory actions on the immune system. There are several pro-inflammatory substances that get upregulated by unhealthy gut microbiota, tumor necrosis factor alpha, Interleukin 1 beta as well as Interleukin 6, and each contributes to a continually escalating out-of-control environment because each inflammatory signal drives ever more inflammation.

Another biochemical imbalance caused by dysbiosis in obesity occurs with the hormone leptin, which is a crucial hormone to the immune system because it's involved with almost every immune cell. An increased level of leptin can cause some immune cells to be increased and other immune cells to be decreased. T-reg cells are inversely correlated with leptin[145] – the higher the level of leptin, the lower the level of T-reg cells. As noted above, T-reg cells regulate the actions of the immune system, consequently, one of the results of low T-reg cells is not enough regulation of the immune system - as in autoimmune problems - which is an over-reacting immune system. The tie-in with obesity looks like this: leptin is a hormone stored in adipose, fatty, tissue; people with higher amounts of fatty tissues have a higher amount of leptin. This increased leptin level causes a decrease in T-reg cell functioning.

Your immune system is very much impacted by the organisms that comprise your gut microbiota. It has repeatedly been seen that disease processes, whether the disease is in the digestive organs or involving organs outside of the digestive organs, many diseases can be traced back to a shift in the organisms in the intestinal tract. Diseases such as inflammatory bowel disease, rheumatoid arthritis, asthma, as just a small example, have all been linked to dysbiosis. "The microbiota which is rich in non-beneficial bacteria, favorably induces the maturation of pro-inflammatory immune cells, leading to uncontrolled inflammation resulting in tissue damage of the mucosal compartment."[146] The damaged cells in the gut mucosa layer then set off a cascade of more inflammatory signals, which progressively results in the immune system failing to control the gut microbiota, which just perpetuates the diseased state.

The bi-directional communication between the gut and the different parts of your immune system is of course necessary in order to sustain life. Healthy microbes in the intestinal tract support health throughout the body and in a healthy state, there is no need for inflammation that is unnecessary, and even counter-productive, such as all chronic inflammatory states. "Gut microbiota interacts with both innate and adaptive immune system, playing a pivotal role in maintenance and disruption of gut immune quiescence"[147] thereby maintaining homeostasis. The two distinct parts of your immune system, the innate and adaptive, are given directions from the gut bacteria on the action they need to take. Like all the research studies presented, there are many more studies claiming the result that a dysbiotic gut sets off inflammatory reactions, which then continues the cycle of inflammation, which continues to fuel more pathogenic bacteria, causing even more inflammation, and on and on the cycle goes.

Another factor in obesity that becomes altered due to unhealthy gut organisms is gut hormonal signaling involving the gastrointestinal/GI hormones. Your gut actually is responsible for producing a number of different hormones related to appetite and other necessary functions. These gastrointestinal hormones are produced by microbes in the mucosa, the innermost layer of the GI tract. It is a fairly new realization that the gut-endocrine system is our largest endocrine system, larger in the scope of how many hormones it makes and the range of diversity of functions these hormones serve in comparison to other endocrine glands. Functions of the gastrointestinal hormones related to food and energy balance include stimulating or decreasing appetite, storing calories or utilizing calories, directing whether fat gets stored or used, directing if insulin gets secreted – these are just some of the functions of the gastrointestinal hormones. Unfortunately, in obesity, the changes to the GI hormones actually drives more weight gain.

A gut microbiota with healthy microbes has a healthy and functioning mucosa that produces appropriate hormonal signals for what the body requires. As already seen in people with obesity, the microbes in the intestinal tract are the types seen in people with disease processes, and those microbes send false signals to the body. In studies comparing different gut-hormone levels between people with obesity and people who are not obese, there are differences. The current thought is these differences are the result of the microbes in the gut, as seen with calorie storage previously.

Leptin has hormonal properties as well as the immune system properties already discussed. When acting as a hormone, leptin plays a key role in stimulation and suppression of appetite. Leptin is the leading signaling molecule in adipose tissue and as such "is a key sensor of energy metabolism and a cornerstone in the regulation of metabolism-immune system interplay."[148] When leptin levels rise, which they do after you eat, they give the message to your brain that you are no longer hungry.

But, obesity leads to hyper-leptin release which results in leptin resistance due to over-stimulation on the leptin receptor sites. The next step in the cascade "is central leptin resistance, caused by impairment of leptin transportation, leptin signaling and leptin target neural circuits,"[149] and "is considered the main risk factor for the obesity pathogenesis."[150] It can be compared with the situation of receiving daily phone calls from solicitors; your solution is to not answer those phone calls – you ignore them. Your body/brain responds the same way with that increased level of leptin, the leptin signaling gets ignored, and that's leptin resistance.

As already seen, leptin levels get disturbed by unhealthy gut bacteria. These alterations cause changes that produce false appetite signals as a result of the leptin resistance. In leptin resistance the brain does not pick up on the signals from the leptin informing the brain that the body has enough calories. Because the brain is not "told" by leptin that the body has enough calories, the person always feels hungry. It is connecting the dots; one problem causes the next which causes the next, and on and on.

Ghrelin is another gastroendocrine hormone playing a cornerstone role in appetite and in how calories get used. Ghrelin is known as the appetite stimulator, but it has another function related to food as well. Ghrelin is involved with decreasing energy output and promotes storage of calories into fat tissue. This function of ghrelin can be viewed as that of conserving calories. More people know of ghrelin as the hormone that makes you feel hungry. Ghrelin levels rise to increase your appetite. Then as you are eating, the ghrelin levels go down since your brain does not need to get the message that you need to eat. Ghrelin and leptin levels are supposed to be opposed to one another, when one is high the other is low, and these levels shift as needed. Ghrelin levels also get altered by a dysbiotic gut, sending out false signals. Studies on people with obesity have shown differences in ghrelin levels compared to people who are not obese. In several studies, ghrelin levels did not decrease as much from eating a meal in obese people compared to people who are not obese.[151] [152] This means that the slightly elevated levels of ghrelin are still sending the message to your brain that your body needs calories, thereby resulting in still feeling hungry, which results in the person continuing to eat more calories than they really need. This occurs at every meal, even at other times throughout the day and night; and this becomes another route that drives a person to consume more calories on a consistent basis than their body needs. These un-needed calories get put into storage, which is fatty tissue, perpetuating the momentum of obesity.

The previous chapter cited a study that put the participants on either an animal food diet or a vegan diet for five days and observed the differences in gut organisms due to the diets. This same study also found changes to metabolic activity from the two distinct diets which is prevalent with regards to obesity and how calories get utilized. From the study, "Analysis of fecal SCFAs (short-chain fatty acids) and bacterial clusters suggests that macronutrient shifts on both diets also altered microbial metabolic activity."[153] In just five days, the foods eaten caused enough of a shift in the microbes living in the gut that there was a noticeable effect on metabolism.

There are many other gut hormones that contribute to whether your appetite is increased or decreased, whether calories get used or stored, whether your blood-glucose levels stay elevated or return to healthy levels following a meal and there are hundreds of studies showing alterations of these gut-hormones in people with obesity. These gastro-endocrine hormones have long names and it gets pretty technical. At this point you have already read the basics and can see clearly the direct cause-and-effect relationship, so we will move on, keeping the knowledge that the organisms in the gut cause the production, lack of production, and over production of each of these gut hormones, all of which have ramifications to the body.

A large number of the hormones produced in the gastroendocrine system are also neurotransmitters that affect your brain. These hormones/neurotransmitters, produced in the gastroendocrine system will be discussed in the section "Your Gut Microbiome and Your Brain."

Studies have seen that it is not completely about the foods you eat, it is also about what organisms are living in your gut that are able to break down and extract the phytonutrients from the foods eaten. Here is the sequence, the foods you eat are the substrate for organisms to develop and then these organisms build the microbiota. But you don't get the healthy health-promoting bacteria without eating vegetables, fruits, grains, nuts, and seeds. This is crucial because some foods inhibit the growth of unhealthy pathogenic bacteria while promoting healthy organisms, contrasted to other foods that actually cause unhealthy pathogenic organisms to develop and cause a cascade of inflammatory processes; there is more detail on this in the earlier chapter "The Western Diet's Influence on the Microbiome," and very specifically with regards to emulsifiers and artificial sweeteners. The phytonutrients are available to your body when the organisms are the healthy organisms and able to pull out those phytonutrients and make them available to your body. But your gut will only have those healthy types of health-promoting organisms if you consistently eat vegetables and fruits more than processed foods or the SAD. The great news is that study after study have shown that by changing to a vegan or vegetarian diet, the organisms in the gut change and the consequence is a change to the overall health.

You are able to choose health. If you want it. The magical wizard is you. What do you want for your future?

Plant Foods Increase Bacterial Diversity

Just like there are studies showing the harmful effects of the SAD to the microbiome, there are studies showing what happens in the human microbiome from eating plant foods. All these studies are eye-opening, some of the results you have already read in this book, and there are more in the next few pages.

Plant foods increase bacterial diversity. Research studies prove that people with a higher intake of plant foods, vegetables, and some fruit have a more diverse bacterial population in their gut. This wide spectrum of healthy strains of bacteria separates health from disease. It makes the difference because it is the organisms in your gut that break down the foods you eat and make the phytonutrients from the foods available to your body. It is also the organisms that either promote anti-inflammatory signaling that keeps inflammation in your body at healthy levels or induces inflammatory events that set the stage for other disease processes to occur. The consequence of having a diversity of healthy microbes is the healthier organisms then function to maintain your health by supplying your body the substances it needs to function optimally while keeping diseases at bay.

High-throughput testing has allowed scientists and researchers to discern the different types of organisms in the gut microbiota, allowing them to see clearly the differences in which types of organisms live in people with disease processes compared with people without those same disease processes. This sheds new light on diseases and how to treat them and more importantly, from my perspective, how to prevent them. Just as you read some of the small amount of information from studies elucidating the causal link between gut microbes and diseases, there are numerous studies depicting the health-promoting effects of microbes. One such study states, "The commensal bacteria appear to be important in suppressing inflammatory response and promoting immunological tolerance, and this interaction also occurs through"[154] receptors on the cells. Immunological tolerance is the ability of your immune system to recognize self-tissues and not mount an attack on those self-tissues. Self-tissues refers to all the different types of tissues that make up your body – your skin, muscles, joints, organs, glands, and central nervous system. Autoimmune disorders are the loss of the immune system's self-tolerance, resulting in tissues getting attacked by the immune system whether it's a gland being attacked or an organ, joints, muscles, skin, or even the central nervous system.

In another study these two authors noted that "The spread of the Western lifestyle has been accompanied by microbial changes thought to underlie the emergence of chronic, nontransmissible, immune-related diseases. The past decade has seen the unprecedented development of therapies for 'replenishing' the microbiota of sick individuals."[155] Never before in history have medical interventions been needed at the rate currently needed just to "replenish," as the authors put it, our microbes that make up our health. They also note, as other researchers have, that a plant-based diet produces a more diverse bacterial environment in the gut. This is very important because the more diversity in the organisms the more efficient those organisms are at preventing pathogenic organisms from colonizing.

A two-week study in Moscow of 248 people also concluded that the people that ate high amounts of plants during this study increased their gut microbes to communities of microbes that were similar to gut microbes seen in people with long-term high plant intakes.[156] Also seen in this study was "A higher intake of vegetables and fruits was associated with increased levels of butyrate-producing *Clostridiales* and higher community richness."[157] (More on butyrate in the section "What's the Deal With Short-chain fatty acids?") Also of note, at the end of the study, the organisms existing in the gut before the start of the dietary changes were then compared to those organisms that were in the gut after the high intake of plants and the researchers found that just the two weeks made "profound changes in community structure"[158] and the changes in the types of organisms is "associated with a higher diversity of diet."[159]

The chapter "Research Links Western Diet to Health Problems" referenced a study where researchers observed children from a rural village in Africa and compared their gut microbiotas with those of children from Europe. The children were between 2-6 years old. The African children had a plant-based diet high in fiber, legumes, and fruit, while the children from Europe had a Western-style diet dominated by animal fat, low fruit, low legumes, and low fiber intake. A richer microbe-filled gut was seen in the African children compared with the European children. The researchers wrote, "the African children exhibited increased richness and biodiversity in their faecal microbiota compared to that identified in European children"[160]

The importance of a diverse gut microbiota cannot be over emphasized. A diverse community of the health-promoting bacteria and other organisms is the body's defense against pathogenic bacteria. It is always about who has the real estate – the good guys or the bad guys. When it comes to staking claim of gut territory, if there are more of the healthy and varied types of bacteria the better their chances of holding ground. Think of this in terms of superheroes going into a battle- really – it's the good guys, the defenders, against the bad guys. If Iron Man, Black Widow, Captain America, Thor, Scarlet Witch, Black Panther and Hawkeye had to battle 20 bad guys, it would end well because these good guys are great at defending their territory. The other huge plus is each of them is skilled at a different mode of defense, adding improved chances for being able to win the battle. But, if these seven superheroes had to fight 400 bad guys, it is going to be a tougher battle even with their wide range of skills. It is the same, and the reality, with regards to the microbes in your intestinal tract – the higher the numbers and the bigger the diversity, the better. The healthy bacteria provide colonization resistance against pathogenic bacteria. Colonization resistance occurs in several ways: microbes competing for nutrients; microbes competing for space in the intestines; the good guys secrete substances that restrain the bad guys; and other factors that involve immune system signaling to participate in the battle.[161] But, if the majority of the organisms in the gut are bad guys, other bad guys more easily colonize.

Another fascinating study on gut diversity revealed its impact on blood vessel health. The title of this study is *Gut microbial diversity is associated with lower arterial stiffness in women,* and it revealed that, "Gut microbiome diversity is inversely associated with arterial stiffness in women."[162] This was the first study in humans to see the correlation between the gut microbiota and its effect on blood vessels, specifically arterial stiffness. It is commonly believed that arterial stiffness occurs with age, and especially with chronic systemic inflammation, but now we can see there is a specific causative factor driving it.

Numerous studies have been cited showing that lack of bacterial diversity is seen in several autoimmune diseases. Some of these diseases are inflammatory bowel disease[163], atopic eczema[164], type 1 diabetes[165], type 2 diabetes[166], psoriatic arthritis[167], obesity[168], and rheumatoid arthritis.[169] Studies have also shown the opposite, that people without those listed disease processes have bacterial diversity.

There was a very interesting study in people with rheumatoid arthritis that showed: "In a single-blind dietary intervention study, 24 patients with moderate-to-severe RA (rheumatoid arthritis) reported significant reductions in symptoms with a four-week, very low-fat (approximately 10%), vegan diet."[170] The results after just four weeks was a significant reduction in weight "and all measures of RA symptomatology decreased significantly ... except for duration of morning stiffness." These were great results! Just think how much better those people could be if they ate a vegan diet, or a mostly vegan diet, for a longer period. As morning stiffness is a hallmark symptom of rheumatoid arthritis there is a chance that it would lessen the longer the person ate a vegan diet high in vegetables.

Another great study, and recommended read, is titled *Plant-Based Dietary Patterns and Incidence of Type 2 Diabetes in US Men and Women: Results from Three Prospective Cohort Studies.* In this study the researchers reviewed three large-scale studies that each took place over many years and reviewed thousands of Americans: "69,949 women from the Nurses' Health Study (1984-2012), 90,239 women from the Nurses' Health Study 2 (1991-2011), and 40,539 men from the Health Professionals Follow-Up Study (1986-2010), free of chronic diseases at baseline."[171] Among these thousands of people, the researchers consistently saw that the people with the higher intake of healthy vegetables and with a healthier BMI did not develop type 2 diabetes. The conclusion written by these researchers was, "Our study suggests that plant-based diets, especially when rich in high-quality plant foods, are associated with substantially lower risk of developing T2D (type 2 diabetes). This supports current recommendations to shift to diets rich in healthy plant foods, with lower intake of less healthy plant and animal foods..." [172]

The common denominator in these two studies, as well as the thousands of others achieving similar results, is the diversity of organisms that develops in the gut microbiota from eating high amounts of plant foods. That cause-and-effect relationship between consuming more plant foods and reaping a more diverse gut microbiota was elucidated earlier in this section.

Numerous studies have discovered that people who live in countries that continue to eat the traditional diet from the past have a much wider range of bacteria in their gut, are dominant in a population of bacteria that people in the US and Europe do not have, and have a lower incidence of autoimmune problems.

One of these studies compared the gut microbiota from two different tribes in Papua New Guinea with the gut microbiota from people in the United States. The two tribes from Papua New Guinea had a higher level of diversity compared to the microbiotas from the people from the United States.[173] The tribes from Papua New Guinea have a plant-based diet. The researchers thought that the differences in lifestyle were the causative force behind the differences seen in these groups of people and stated, "that westernization may decrease bacterial dispersal rates, altering microbiota structure."[174]

A standout study on a group of people from the Amazon achieved drastically different results compared to results from studies thus far. This group of people from a Yanomami Ameridian village has remained mostly isolated for more than 11,000 years and are still hunter-gatherers following the traditional lifestyle of their ancestors. This study characterized the microbiotas of their intestines, mouth and skin and discovered "the highest diversity of bacteria and genetic functions ever reported in a human group."[175] Comparatively, "The study showed that the Ameridians harbor a highly diverse microbiome when compared with western US and Italians, agrarian Malawi and Guahibo populations, and hunter-gatherer populations of Tanzania, with the highest gut diversity found this far."[176]

Raw unprocessed foods provide our bodies with a variety of bacteria because their phytonutrients are nutrients that health-promoting bacteria need. Therefore, consuming raw unprocessed foods is one way to acquire diverse and health-promoting bacteria. These foods affect the human microbiome in the positive way we need, fueling a healthy intestinal microbiota. When food gets processed, of course all the types of bacteria get eliminated and we do not develop any healthful bacteria from that processed food. This is the same thing that happens when we take antibiotics. When we take an antibiotic it wipes out numerous types of bacteria, sickness-causing bacteria types and health-promoting necessary bacteria. The antibiotic is non-discriminating in exactly the same way as foods that are processed.

Cooked vegetables also provide our bodies with the phytonutrients they need, and have a positive effect on our microbiome due to the organisms that develop from their indigestible fibers. When cooking vegetables, steaming, but only to the point of becoming a bright color, is a good method. Vegetables should never be steamed to the point of losing their color and becoming mushy. Roasting, sautéing, and blanching are also good methods of cooking vegetables.

Plant foods contain indigestible fiber, which is the substrate for developing short-chain fatty acids (SCFAs), which are prebiotic for your intestinal tract. (More on SCFAs in the section "What's the Deal With Short-chain fatty acids?") Prebiotics refers to substances that cannot get digested and are the substrate that promote the development of healthy organisms in the intestines. Most people know about probiotics which are healthy strains of bacteria and yeasts, which should be living in the gut microbiota. Prebiotics instead are the substrates healthy bacteria develop from. Plant foods are prebiotic. Consuming fiber every day is vital to a healthy microbiome and intestinal microbiota.

The Gut Microbiota and Your Brain

It's time to discuss the gut-brain axis.

"The what-what-who? Run that by me again." You might be asking, "How is brain chemistry affected by the intestinal microbiota?"

First, consider that your gut is commonly referred to as your second brain, and rightly so because there are 500 million neurons that communicate from your gut to your brain; this is five times more neurons than from the spinal cord to your brain! Very important is the fact that communication is bi-directional – your brain communicates to your gut what is going on and your gut communicates to your brain what is going on in the gut. Think about it, how do you know when you are hungry? Is it because you feel it in your stomach? And, if you feel it in your stomach, how does that message get to your brain? If your stomach couldn't communicate with your brain, you would not know you were hungry. (This is the reality of all mechanisms in the body, there must be two-way communication. Without it, bodily functions and processes would not get started, turned off, or slowed down. All processes in the human body are a result of feed-back loops.)

There are three distinct systems in the body that are routes of communication in the gut-brain axis. One of those routes is via hormones and neurotransmitters, which are signaling agents that are released in one part of the body and then cause an action in a different part of the body. There are hundreds of these in your gut that communicate with your brain. The second route of communication is neural, where the vagus nerve communicates between your gut and your brain. The third communication system is the immune system.

The communication network of the gut-brain axis is vital to your life, pointing to the need for overlap among these systems, or redundancy, the backup for the backup. Redundancy in the body serves as a safety mechanism ensuring that important jobs get done.

The first route we will discuss is via hormones and neurotransmitters that communicate between your gut and your brain. Surprisingly, there are more neuronal connections between your gut and your brain then there are between your spine and your brain. Another fascinating fact regarding neurotransmitters/hormones and your gut – your gut secretes more neurotransmitters/hormones than any other single endocrine gland![177] The other endocrine glands secrete one or just a few hormones. This makes your gut the largest endocrine gland in your body. As one group of researchers put it, "it is far larger and more biochemically heterogeneous than any other endocrine organ."[178] Currently it appears that much of the hormonal communication between the gut and brain is through the Hypothalamus-Pituitary-Adrenal axis, or HPA axis, which relies on neurotransmitters and hormones to be made in appropriate amounts. This communication impacts the hypothalamus which then stimulates the anterior pituitary which then causes stimulation to the adrenals, resulting in either production of cortisol or suppression of cortisol. In simpler terms, the bacteria in your intestines affect the HPA axis and cause cortisol release or suppression. Cortisol release in your body causes you to feel "stressed".

There are many studies proving that stress will cause a change in the organisms in the gut, and there are also studies showing that it is the gut organisms that increase the stress response. Connect this to the fact that all communication between the brain and gut is bi-directional - meaning that the organisms in the gut have direct effect into the brain and brain activity has a direct effect on the environment of the gut. Think about this reaction for a moment: if unhealthy organisms in the gut are causing a heightened stress response resulting in an increased cortisol, which causes more systemic inflammation and immune system suppression, which then allows the unhealthy organisms in the gut to thrive, this becomes a self-perpetuating cycle. Just to be clear, the changes stress makes in the organisms in the gut consistently cause an increase in unhealthy bacteria, but never do they increase the healthy types of bacteria.

Some of the hormones involved in the communication between the brain and the gut were discussed in the section "Research Links Western Diet to Health Problems." We already discussed some of the hormones involved in appetite, or calorie usage or storage, but, there are many more hormones and neurotransmitters that are crucial to optimal functioning of the body that are produced by organisms in the gut and communicate to the brain. In fact, your gut uses more than 30 neurotransmitters that are identical to neurotransmitters found in your brain. These neurotransmitters affect how you think and how you feel. Some of the hormones do double duty and also act as neurotransmitters, such as serotonin, dopamine, and norepinephrine. The neurotransmitters that are in your gut and influence your brain include serotonin, dopamine, norepinephrine, glutamate, acetylcholine, and nitric oxide along with others. The production of serotonin, dopamine, norepinephrine and acetylcholine takes place in the intestinal tract and requires certain types of bacteria. Each of these neurotransmitters requires specific bacteria to break down certain foods in order to produce these specific neurotransmitters. Changes in bacterial species change the production of these neurotransmitters as well as others not listed. It has been known that your gut uses upwards of 30 neurotransmitters that are also used in your brain, and now it has been learned that different bacteria alter which and how much of these neurotransmitters get produced. Healthy strains of bacteria produce the amounts of neurotransmitters needed to think clearly, be happy, have stable moods, sleep well as well as other functions. But, unhealthy strains of bacteria produce an imbalance of the neurotransmitters which negatively impacts your brain, your functioning and well being.

Let's use serotonin as an example since much is known about its functions and it is essential to your brain and in regulating your intestinal tract also. The majority of your serotonin, 90%, is actually found in your bowels and not the brain. This may be surprising to you since most people know that serotonin levels are thought to correlate with depression which is naturally thought to be an issue of the brain; and serotonin is the key neurotransmitter that is low in people with depression.

So, the next question would be, "Where do we get our serotonin from?" Your gut! Serotonin is made by specific organisms in your gut from tryptophan. Certain bacteria transform tryptophan into serotonin, but if those specific bacteria are relatively low in numbers the conversion into serotonin would also be low. Most depression has everything to do with the gut microbiota.

Here is an interesting correlation: depression is seen often enough in patients with irritable bowel syndrome/IBS and inflammatory bowel disease/IBD that even before science knew about the different microorganisms in the gut, the very high incidence indicated there had to be a relationship. Depression is considered a co-morbidity with IBS patients. And now we know that most depression is a result of a gut microbiota that houses unhealthy organisms that are not capable of making serotonin in the amounts needed for optimal mental health. (This is a simplistic view as other neurotransmitters such as dopamine, epinephrine and acetylcholine also are involved.)

Depression is also seen as a co-morbidity with insomnia. Your sleep is also directly impacted by the organisms in your gut microbiota, as it is the HPA axis that plays a critical role in sleep. When it comes to sleep, it is a multi-hormonal event. Some of the hormones involved in getting and staying asleep are serotonin, insulin, cortisol, norepinephrine, dopamine, and acetylcholine, some of which need to be elevated and some decreased for sleep to occur. Basically, the same list of hormones seen above that are produced in the gut by certain bacteria need to be produced in the correct amounts in order for good quality sleep. Hmmmmm. "Interesting, so you're telling me, if I have the healthy types of bacteria in my gut I will have better moods, and better sleep?" The answer is yes!

One more very common health problem that shares some of those same hormonal alterations is anxiety. As stated just a few paragraphs earlier, a gut microbiota with unhealthy bacteria has definitively been proven to cause a heightened stress response. Once again a correlation among people with IBS and IBD and what is thought of as a brain issue has been noticed. Doctors and gastroenterologists have observed a high incidence of anxiety among their patients with IBS and IBD. This is directly due to the microbes in the gut and whether they are converting tryptophan to serotonin, which is involved with sleep, depression, and anxiety. To this point, a group of research scientists discovered from stool samples from IBD patients that they all had less capacity for metabolizing tryptophan.[179]

This is a very simplistic view of depression, insomnia, and anxiety as it focuses on just serotonin. There are other neurotransmitters that play a role in these conditions that are also not produced in correct amounts in a dysbiotic gut. The neurotransmitters that are produced in too-high or too- low levels cause a cascade of events that lead to depression, insomnia, anxiety, and other moods and behaviors. A study done on germ-free mice determined "that the vast majority of chemicals circulating in blood are dependent on the microbiome for their synthesis, although many are subsequently modified by the host."[180]

"These chemicals have a profound effect on mammalian behavior and neuroendocrine responses."[181]

There are many other hormonal cascades that occur from the other hormones/neurotransmitters mentioned, and there are many others not mentioned, so this section only gave you the view of serotonin. Keep in mind there are many hormonal effects that are directly impacted by your gut microbiota. With my patients I often explain this as a domino effect: in the body when just one of the hormones/neurotransmitters is not being produced in the correct amount it will cause changes affecting the other hormones/neurotransmitters.

The subject of hormones/neurotransmitters is highly technical, and will not be discussed further in this book. So next we'll take a look at how the vagus nerve is involved in the communication between the brain and the gut.

The second route of communication between the gut and brain is via the vagus nerve. The vagus nerve performs several jobs in its communication to the brain. One of its main jobs is to serve as the conduit between your gut and your brain. In this capacity, approximately 80% of the vagus nerve function is to communicate from your gut to your brain, the other 20% of the vagus nerve connection travels in the opposite direction from your brain to your gut. (Your liver, heart and lungs are also in constant communication with your brain via the vagus nerve.)

Some of the communication between the gut and your brain regards inflammatory signaling. The vagus nerve signals to dampen down inflammation in the gut as long as the healthy types of bacteria and organisms are present which do not live in, thrive in, an inflammatory state. By maintaining a non-inflamed intestinal environment, this gut environment is conducive for healthy organisms to thrive whereas the inflamed gut is conducive for unhealthy organisms to thrive in.

The vagus nerve is also responsible for decreasing intestinal permeability. The intestinal tract needs to remain non-permeable to foods and other types of cells in order to avoid health problems, as seen in IBS, IBD, colitis, and Crohn's disease. A permeable intestinal tract allows foods and other cells to escape the intestines which should not be outside of the intestines, causing systemic inflammatory reactions. Recall that the intestines is supposed to be an encased tube that only permits contents to enter from the upper end and exit through the lower opening. The inflamed intestinal environment is commonly termed "leaky gut syndrome" precisely because food particles do escape the intestines which then manifests as a person experiencing reactions to certain foods. These reactions are usually gas, bloating, and intestinal pain.

As noted earlier, the vagus nerve can either inhibit or activate inflammation depending on the signals it receives from the organisms in the gut. It actually responds differently to healthy microbes than unhealthy microbes. The vagus nerve response from healthy microbes sets off signals to stop inflammation, while stimulation from unhealthy microbes sets off signals to the immune system to create inflammation. The vagus nerve response from pathogenic organisms also causes increased intestinal permeability – as just mentioned, another of the functions of the vagus nerve to the gut is to keep the cells of the intestines in a non-permeable state. Now think about the compound effects of just these two details to the large intestines. Unhealthy organisms send a signal to cause inflammation in the gut and this signal also causes a loss of structural integrity to the intestines so it becomes permeable – which will result in more immune system activation – so yet another self-perpetuating cycle.

There is more information coming up regarding the inflammation that occurs as a result of pathogenic organisms, but make a mental note that the inflammation happens from immune system activity.

The other main job of the vagus nerve is as the main nerve communicating to the parasympathetic nervous system. The parasympathetic nervous system is the balance to the sympathetic nervous system. Most people know about the sympathetic nervous system, which prepares us for fight-or-flight to physically take on stressful situations, like a bear attack. The sympathetic nervous system biochemically prepares you to get into action. The parasympathetic nervous system does mostly the opposite, it is the calming part of your nervous system that allows you to go to sleep, relax, be creative, all things you would do when not in a stressful situation. As long as the vagus nerve is sending the correct signals to the brain, your parasympathetic nervous system can be dominating and you can be calm, focus, fall asleep and other life-sustaining functions.

The vagus nerve responds to physical stimulus as well as the neurotransmitters, which are biochemical in nature. The vagus nerve activates the HPA axis/Hypothalamus-Pituitary-Adrenal axis, getting the body ready to address a stressful situation in a nano-second if need be. As this is its role, it is always involved in all stress situations. Even chronic stress causes an activation of the HPA axis through the vagus nerve biochemically as well as physically. A very important point to note here is that chronic systemic inflammation puts your body in stress mode; thus, chronic systemic inflammation activates the vagus nerve by activating the HPA axis. Even if you aren't consciously feeling stressed, background chronic systemic inflammation can be present and does have your body in a stressed state.

Serotonin is a biochemical stimulant to the vagus nerve. The result from serotonin signaling to the vagus nerve is to induce the parasympathetic nervous system, creating a calming relaxed state. Serotonin must be produced in order for this specific cascade of signaling to take place. As written earlier, serotonin is made from certain microbes. Without those specific microbes, serotonin does not get made in adequate amounts, which means the vagus nerve does not get signaled by it to induce the parasympathetic nervous system.

The third route of communication between your gut and your brain is through the immune system. I'm sure everyone would easily agree that your immune system has to be in communication with your brain, right? That is an easy one. But, once you stop to think about why it is necessary for the immune system to have a presence in the gut and that those immune cells must also be able to communicate with the brain, it shows you the complex reality that is our amazing human body. Your immune system needs to know what is happening in your intestinal tract as this is the interface of the external world (foods) into your internal world (GI tract/interior) of your body. The role of your immune system in your gut is to inform your immune system if pathogenic bacteria or other organisms or something toxic has been ingested. As soon as that information is relayed to the immune system, there is an immune reaction against that problem to eliminate it as fast as possible. An example is the reaction to food poisoning, where a food delivers large amount of harmful organisms into the body. Your immune system reacts by causing vomiting to expel the dangerous organisms as fast as possible. Makes sense right?

Your vagus nerve has a multitude of neural connections throughout your intestinal tract connecting your brain with what is called the neuro-endocrine axis. This neural network is your first-line defense in the event of ingested pathogens, chemicals, or other harmful substances. If a harmful substance has been ingested this neural network tells your immune system, which quickly goes into action by secreting a temporary inflammatory response through a few inflammatory pathways. This inflammation is only supposed to be a temporary reaction to address an acute situation. Built into this communication that spurs on the inflammation is also a feedback loop to then stop the inflammation once an appropriate amount has already been produced. Again, this is evidence of the wisdom in the human body. This is vital because if inflammation continues unchecked, it causes other problems.

These are just the basics of the vagus neuro-endocrine immune response without getting into technical terms. Even through the introduction of these basics you can see the overlap between the three major systems that communicate between your gut and your brain-hormones/neurotransmitters; vagus nerve; and immune system. Just as pointed out above, this redundancy is critical as it ensures that important jobs get done.

So, let's put this together, healthy organisms in the gut are the catalysts for serotonin production. Serotonin is then the catalyst to create a calm relaxed state. Serotonin in correct proportions counteracts being in an anxiety state. Serotonin in correct proportions give you the ability to fall asleep. At the same time, that serotonin keeps your intestines in a healthy non-inflamed and non-permeable state. This is an environment in which healthy organisms thrive and, as such, they band together in warding off unhealthy organisms. Concurrently, healthy organisms create signaling to the neuro-endocrine system, which dampens down inflammation and signals to not create it.

Contrast the above scenario to unhealthy organisms, which manifests as low or no serotonin, translating to the vagus nerve not getting the correct message and then not stimulating the parasympathetic nervous system. The effect from that is not being able to get into a relaxed state or being able to fall asleep. At the same time the body is under a stress response set off by the unhealthy organisms. This stressed state stimulates the vagus to stimulate the HPA axis which induces more stress hormones and neurotransmitters fueling the stress response even more. This stress response causes changes into the gut microbiota allowing unhealthy types of organisms to thrive. Concurrent with these actions, the neuro-endocrine system is alerted by the opportunistic pathogenic organisms to create inflammation, which causes the intestines to become permeable creating the perfect environment for unhealthy microbes to thrive as each of these actions perpetuates the cycle of inflammation and intestinal permeability.

It now makes sense that IBS and IBD patients who have

dysbiosis commonly have hormonal alterations manifesting in depression, anxiety, and insomnia, as seen above.

In another very informative report researchers concluded that studies on patients with liver cirrhosis and short bowel syndrome saw enough pathological changes to their brains that they could "speculate on possible adverse effects of gut microbes in alcohol dependence, CFS (chronic fatigue syndrome), fibromyalgia, RLS (restless leg syndrome), ASD (autism spectrum disorder), schizophrenia, mood disorders, and degenerative or autoimmune neurologic disease."[182] They had noted negative effects to the central nervous system that were "attributed to alterations in bacterial community structure (dysbiosis), SIBO (small intestinal bacterial overgrowth), and increased intestinal permeability."[183]

Another health crisis all people would like to avoid is Alzheimer's disease and Parkinson's disease, there is such a strong correlation between Alzheimer's and Parkinson's with digestive disorders that the disorders are seen as co-morbidities to these brain function diseases.[184] [185] [186] Chronic digestive disorders all share multiple factors that drive chronic inflammation affecting neurotransmitters, hormones and several other factors that become negatively impacted. Each of these factors drive more dis-ease throughout the body and brain, taking the body farther and farther away from a healthy state. A key factor here in effecting your brain function is the fact that chronic systemic inflammation causes changes to the blood-brain barrier rendering it more permeable. We've discussed how the intestinal barrier is negatively affected by pathogenic microbes, but we did not review the fact that chronic systemic inflammation also alters the blood brain barrier. The blood brain barrier's job is to closely regulate which substances can come in and out of your brain, protecting your brain from substances that could negatively affect the structures and functioning while retaining what it needs. An increased permeability allows nutrients and other molecules to cross into the brain which otherwise should not be, thereby affecting brain activity and brain health.

There are numerous scientific studies from different groups of researchers that concluded that digestive disorders played a role in later developing neuro-degenerative diseases such as Alzheimer's and Parkinson's. This is a hot-topic for researchers due to the increasing numbers of people experiencing neuro-degenerative diseases and, since there is no effective cure, prevention is the best course of action. Also, now due to technological advances, scientists are now able to see the clear cause-effect relationship between the gut microbiota and neuro-degenerative diseases. It is clear to many scientists that the different types of organisms in people's gut microbiotas are affecting organs and causing health problems, which then affect the brain.

Alzheimer's disease (AD) is the number one neuro-degenerative disease. In a comparative study of the organisms from the guts from people with Alzheimer's contrasted with people that do not have Alzheimer's, these researchers wrote: "Our analyses revealed that the gut microbiome of AD participants has decreased microbial diversity and is compositionally distinct from control age- and sex-matched individuals."[187] Additionally, these researchers saw links between the abundant types of organisms and markers for Alzheimer's in the cerebral spinal fluid.[188] "These findings add AD to the growing list of diseases associated with gut microbial alterations,"[189] they stated.

A different study enrolled 1,646 people and the researchers concluded "We report for the first time an association between altered BA (bile acid) profile, genetic variants implicated in AD and cognitive changes in disease using a large multicenter study. These findings warrant further investigation of gut dysbiosis and possible role of gut liver brain axis in the pathogenesis of AD."[190] This is just a small example of current research proving the correlation between gut health and brain health. There are other numerous studies that have had similar findings, and they are amazing and eye opening if you care to do an internet search. If more people knew this, I believe more people would take control of their health and their brain.

Parkinson's disease (PD) is also of great concern as it is the second leading neuro-degenerative disease. Here are some statements from researchers from different studies regarding Parkinson's disease and gut health.

In this study the group of researchers compared the gut microbiota of people with Parkinson's disease to the gut microbiota of people without Parkinson's disease. The groups were age and sex matched. The details in this study are fascinating. They showed there were distinct differences in the gut bacterial compositions between these two groups. The people with Parkinson's disease had increased amounts of a few different groups of organisms that cause inflammation, and did not have the same groups and types of organisms that were present in the people without Parkinson's disease.[191] The people without Parkinson's disease had bacterial strains that did not promote inflammation.[192] These researchers concluded with this: "This report provides evidence that proinflammatory dysbiosis is present in PD patients and could trigger inflammation-induced misfolding of α-Syn and development of PD pathology."[193] One more fascinating fact is the *Bacteroides* type of gram-negative bacteria that are seen in abundance in Parkinson's disease patients are also seen in abundance in people with type 2 diabetes.[194]

Another group of researchers wrote this: "It has become increasingly evident in recent years that Parkinson's disease is a multicentric neurodegenerative process that affects several neuronal structures outside the substantia nigra, among which is the enteric nervous system."[195] The enteric nervous system is the group of neurons that governs the gastrointestinal tract.

While another group of researchers discovered these findings: "Recent reports have shown that the lesions in the enteric nervous system occur in very early stages of the disease, even before the involvement of the central nervous system. This has led to the postulation that the enteric nervous system could be critical in the pathophysiology of Parkinson's disease, as it could represent the point of entry for a putative environmental factor to initiate the pathological process."[196]

Other researchers, through their experiment on actual patients with Parkinson's disease, stated: "Our data show that our PD subjects exhibit significantly greater intestinal permeability (gut leakiness) than controls. In addition, this intestinal hyperpermeability significantly correlated with increased intestinal mucosa staining for E. coli bacteria,"[197] as well as other factors. "These data represent not only the first demonstration of abnormal intestinal permeability in PD subjects but also the first correlation of increased intestinal permeability in PD with intestinal alpha-synuclein (the hallmark of PD), as well as staining for gram negative bacteria and tissue oxidative stress."[198] You could make the connection here from information you read in the chapter "The Western Diet's Influence on the Microbiome". Recall from the chapter "The Western Diet's Influence on the Microbiome" studies on emulsifiers saw the increase in E. coli migration across intestinal cells due to emulsifiers in processed foods. The researchers in the PD study referenced in this paragraph found actual PD patients have, gut leakiness and increased levels of E coli., so while there is not a definitive answer pointing to emulsifiers causing PD, there is a possible connection. As you can see from all you have read thus far in this book, the body is very complex and even if emulsifiers are involved in the gut leakiness and abundance of E coli. existence, there are probably other contributing factors.

Many scientific studies have been performed on patients with Alzheimer's disease as well as Parkinson's disease that all concluded that there was an increase in the many inflammatory cytokines in these patients. In case you want to know which biomarkers those cytokines are, here are those details: In Alzheimer's disease an increase in IL-6, TNFα, IL-1β, TGFβ, IL-12 and IL-18 is seen.[199] While in Parkinson's disease an increase in IL-6, TNFα, IL-1β, IL-2, IL-10, C-reactive protein and RANTES (regulated on activation, normal T-expressed, and presumably secreted).[200] As you can see, this is not just as simple as "Oh, you have a little chronic inflammation." There are several pathways involved that we know of currently.

One more factor to be aware of is type 3 diabetes, which some researchers are calling Alzheimer's disease. This cognitive function disorder occurs when neurons in the brain become unable to respond to insulin, whether due to insulin resistance or insulin deficiency. Just like insulin in your body carries glucose into the cells as fuel for the cells, it is insulin in the brain that allows brain cells to utilize glucose, which is needed at a very high rate by the cells of the brain. Every action in the brain requires glucose, even basic tasks including memory and learning. Without glucose getting into cells, cells die, brain neurons die, oxidative stress increases, and the hallmark signs of tau-tangles, and amyloid beta plaques ensue - both are primary markers of Alzheimer's. Research shows that type 3 diabetes and type 2 diabetes are both syndromes that are "unequivocally accompanied by significant activation of inflammatory mediators, oxidative stress, DNA damage, and mitochondrial dysfunction, which contribute to the degenerative cascade by exacerbating insulin/IGF (insulin growth factor) resistance."[201]

Type 3 diabetes as a disease is relatively new; some medical professionals are not yet on board with it. Since type 3 diabetes is being considered a type of Alzheimer's disease there are facts to keep in mind with regards to Alzheimer's disease: 1) People with type 2 diabetes have more than 60% increased risk of getting Alzheimer's disease. Though not everyone with diabetes gets Alzheimer's disease, and not everyone with Alzheimer's disease has type 2 diabetes. 2) Type 3 diabetes is most likely a lifestyle disease. Researchers have pointed out that exercise and diet play a critical role in prevention. There is a genetic component involved for some people, but again not every person with Alzheimer's disease has that genetic predisposition. 3) The comment from researchers who saw in both type 2 diabetes and type 3 diabetes that there is "significant activation of inflammatory mediators, oxidative stress, DNA damage, and mitochondrial dysfunction, which contribute to the degenerative cascade by exacerbating insulin/IGF (insulin growth factor) resistance."[202] Both disease processes have multiple biochemical cascades that are perturbed and since, at this point, there is not a clear timeline of what came first no one can say if these unhealthy changes preceded insulin resistance or insulin deficiency. But, you can take cues from the above information on Alzheimer's and Parkinson's that there are first unhealthy microbes that cause changes in biochemical signaling which result in inflammation and if that has been going on for years it continues setting off more dramatic changes in hormones and neurotransmitters, which continually affects the liver, heart, and of course the brain.

Once again, you can connect the dots to see cause and effect: digestive disorders alter the levels of hormones and neurotransmitters changing brain function, pair this with systemic chronic inflammation which changes the blood-brain barrier and you can see how this can lead to bigger problems regarding brain health. Think about these alterations in hormones, neurotransmitters, and from chronic inflammation and you can see the effect they could have over the course of years to the body and the brain. Over the course of years other body systems are progressively affected, altered, and brought farther away from proper functioning while progressing into an unhealthy state. A person experiencing IBS will only continue to progress into worsening states of IBS unless something is done to alter that course. Likewise with the other digestive disorders discussed. The changes to the body from IBS will continue to have a negative impact to the other organs, glands, and tissues, causing additional diagnoses of more problems unless changes are made to the microbiome to stop the dis-ease progress.

The numerous beneficial effects from vegetables for our overall health and long-term brain health is due to several factors: 1) phytonutrients, 2) fiber, 3) vital help to the mitochondria from the phytonutrients, 4) someone eating a lot of vegetables most likely is not eating much processed foods. If they are not hungry because they have eaten vegetables, the tank is full, unless that person over-eats.

Your Microbiome Affects Your Liver and Your Liver Affects Your Microbiome

In the past 10 years technology has allowed researchers to look into relationships in the human body in ways that were previously not possible. The ability to discern some of the many different organisms in the gut has been groundbreaking and has brought us a different view of our reality. This view is also allowing us to see how the different types of organisms cause biochemical reactions as well as allowing researchers to look deeper at the relationships and influences among distinct organs due to organisms.

We'll first look at liver health and how it impacts the brain, and then we'll look at the effect the gut microbiota has on the liver. Many studies have seen proof of how the liver affects the brain and how the gut microbiota, the intestines, influence the health of the liver.

Here is as brief a description of what your liver does as can be written. The liver may actually have more than 500 functions to perform. These are functions no other organ can do, which is why you cannot live without a liver. All these crucial jobs help maintain homeostasis. They are:

Blood detoxification and purification: Your liver is the organ that removes toxic chemicals, such as drugs and man-made chemicals in processed foods. Your liver excretes the broken-down metabolites of drugs that need to be eliminated as they could be fatal. Your liver also eliminates other toxins, such as waste products from foreign organisms; and old or damaged cells, hormones, and other biochemicals that have already done their job and need to be eliminated as they are no longer useful to your body. Without this function, your body would be overloaded with even just one of these listed categories.

Metabolism of fats, proteins, and carbohydrates: Blood filled with semi-digested food is carried to the liver via the hepatic portal vein from the spleen, pancreas, and small intestines. In this role the liver is the gatekeeper, as everything that has been ingested has to pass through the liver first before it can get into the main blood circulation. The liver is responsible for breaking apart and converting these semi-digested molecules into molecules your cells can use for fuel, or for protein structures in cells, or putting usable forms into storage to be used later.

Excretion of bilirubin and cholesterol: Your liver excretes bilirubin, a waste product from old red blood cells that is toxic to your brain if not excreted. Your liver excretes cholesterol in order to maintain a healthy range of blood cholesterol.

Bile production and excretion: Your liver produces bile to

assist in the breakdown of fats and excretes that bile into the small intestines when fat is eaten.

Storage of glycogen, vitamins, and minerals: Your liver stores carbohydrates in the form of glycogen. When your blood sugar/blood glucose levels fall, the glycogen is converted to the usable form of glucose and carried into the blood stream to be used by the cells. Your liver also stores vitamins and minerals for future on-demand need.

Synthesis of plasma proteins, such as albumin, and clotting factors: Your liver produces the protein albumin that is necessary to keep fluid in the blood vessels and prevent it from leeching out of the blood vessels into tissues, which causes swelling. This is a crucial function. Also, clotting factors are produced by your liver, without which we could bleed to death from an injury.

When we think of the liver breaking down substances it is the mitochondria that actually get this job done. Mitochondria is an organelle in your cells. Your liver has a large number of mitochondria in each liver cell. Each liver cell has between 2,000-4,000 mitochondria, making up about 25% of each cell. (Only the heart has more mitochondria at about 5,000 per cell making up about 40% of each cell.) This large number of mitochondria in the liver is required because the mitochondria have the primary function of producing adenosine triphosphate (ATP). ATP is the fuel source for every cell in your body. ATP supplies cells with energy to perform the jobs they need to do, as well as to fuel the cells themselves for their own maintenance. ATP is the required currency without which there is no life for mammals. ATP is used by every cell, every muscle, and your brain for every action, even thoughts. Think about it as a barter system -

it is the price paid for every action your body takes. Liver cells have a high demand for energy, meaning ATP, to be able to get all the jobs done that are required for your body. The health of your liver is a consequence of the health of the mitochondria which is why the mitochondria are so important.

The mitochondria perform several other vital jobs. When stated above that the liver breaks down drugs, alcohol, and chemicals including man-made chemicals in processed foods, it is actually the mitochondria in the liver that does this work. The mitochondria also make the potent and required enzymes for the process of detoxifying harmful substances, and harmful reactive oxygen species, or ROS. When mitochondria become defective or diminish in numbers it adversely affects health. The result is less ATP production for energy; less detoxifying enzymes which results in an increase in ROS that cause cellular damage; and a reduction in clearing of drugs and chemicals from the body that circulate through the bloodstream affecting all other organs including the brain. "Most forms of chronic liver diseases are associated with the accumulation of damaged mitochondria responsible for abnormal reactive oxygen species (ROS) formation, glutathione (GSH) depletion, protein alkylation, and respiratory complex alterations."[203]

You can see how necessary it is to have functioning mitochondria, but the mitochondria need some protection, and that comes via melatonin. As discussed in a previous section, serotonin is made from specific bacteria in the intestinal tract. Another very important piece of our hormonal puzzle comes in to play through the action of serotonin being a precursor for melatonin. Melatonin is made from serotonin, so if there is not enough serotonin, there cannot be enough melatonin production. Making the connection here, if there is not enough serotonin there will not be enough melatonin to protect the mitochondria in the liver resulting in chemicals, medications and old biochemicals building up in the body. This is just one of the cascades in which intestinal health impacts liver health.

Melatonin has several jobs that are crucial to your health. Most people know of melatonin in relationship to helping sleep but, its most important job is as a very powerful free radical scavenger. Another one of its important jobs is the regulation of the day-night circadian rhythms, which relates to melatonin's ability to promote sleep. Other jobs include immune system homeostasis, regeneration of bone growth, effects mood, anti-inflammatory effects, neuroprotection, and regulation of hormone release. The discovery about melatonin protecting mitochondria is a fairly new discovery. You just read how crucial mitochondria are for your body, and now with this new discovery we learned even more about how vital melatonin is for us because it is what protects the mitochondria. As you see, melatonin is indispensable in its jobs of overseeing an array of physiological, regulatory, and protective functions that have influence throughout your body. And now you understand why melatonin is so important for your liver health and how it affects your brain.

Let's tie this together. It is a known fact that Alzheimer's patients usually have sleep disorders. It is also known that Alzheimer's patients have a high rate of intestinal problems, as discussed in the previous chapter. You also read in the previous chapter, neurotransmitters and hormones get altered as a consequence of digestive disorders, serotonin often becoming impacted, leading to the depression, anxiety and insomnia that are very commonly seen in people with digestive problems. Now, think about the fact that if serotonin is chronically at low levels, how is melatonin supposed to get made? So, the sleep disorders very common among Alzheimer's patients could most likely be one of the manifestations of low melatonin and low serotonin. It is a known fact that Alzheimer's patients have low levels of melatonin. Parkinson's disease patients also commonly have sleep disorders.

But here is one more very important correlation to make regarding the low levels of melatonin and Alzheimer's patients. It is now known that melatonin has anti-amyloid effects preventing amyloid plaques from forming in the brain.[204] [205] [206] That is another crucial protective benefit from melatonin. Remember, amyloid plaques are a hallmark feature of Alzheimer's disease.

One more very crucial connection: the highest amount of melatonin found in the body is in the mitochondria, and your liver is supposed to have high levels of mitochondria. Both Alzheimer's and Parkinson's patients do not produce mitochondria at the rate seen in people of the same age without these diseases.[207] [208] Both Alzheimer's and Parkinson's patients have a high amount of oxidative stress in their brains upon autopsy. [209] [210] Let's take a bio-chemical look at the combined functions of melatonin for the brain: it inhibits amyloid plaque, it's a very powerful antioxidant; and it protects mitochondria so it can continue making ATP to fuel the cells in the brain. Now you can see a clear picture of three factors that are all present in brains of Alzheimer's patients - amyloid plaques, high levels of oxidative damage, and reduced

ATP.

As of this writing the world is in the midst of the COVID19 pandemic, completely new experience to almost everyone, save for the few people still alive who also lived during the 1918 flu. Four months into this pandemic, there was research showing that melatonin levels might actually be one of the crucial factors with regards to how well a person was able to deal with COVID19. Melatonin levels are highest when we are young, then continually decline as we age. The other jobs of melatonin are immune system homeostasis, regeneration of bone growth, effects mood, anti-inflammatory effects, neuroprotection, and regulation of hormone release.

Immune homeostasis is regulated by melatonin, and here's an example: Immune system over-reaction is what caused the cytokine storm in COVID19 patients that led to a large number of deaths. (There are other factors that contributed to other fatal outcomes as this corona virus is a very aggressive virus that attacks the lungs, kidneys, heart, brain and intestines.) People with lower levels of melatonin are usually those who have IBS, IBD, Crohn's Disease, depression, alcoholic fatty liver, elevated liver enzymes due to medications, diabetes, metabolic syndrome, or people that have been on medications for a number of years as there are a number of categories of medications that are known to cause mitochondrial toxicity and consequentially this has a negative effect to the melatonin.

The liver's effect to your brain is eye-opening, as is the effect of the gut microbiota to your liver. If this is new information, it reads like a great Sci-Fi story. Literally, bacteria and their waste products trans-locate to the liver from the intestinal tract and, over the course of years, cause health problems to your liver. While researching on PubMed (https://pubmed.ncbi.nlm.nih.gov/) for "gut microbiota/liver health" at the time of this writing there was 20,845 results (and by the time you read this there will most likely be even more studies.)

From the intestines blood is routed to the liver through the hepatic portal vein. This blood has the absorbed nutrients from semi-digested food and also carries toxins and medications from the intestinal tract to the liver. Studies have shown the liver is affected by bacteria and fungi in people with unhealthy bacterial and fungal overgrowths in the intestinal tract. These pathogenic organisms do trans-locate from the intestines to the liver and then cause problems to the liver, which cumulatively can contribute to damaging and reducing the number of mitochondria. The reduction in mitochondria will cause an increase in the ROS, which will cause not just liver problems but also problems throughout your body impacting your brain and other organs. If the numbers of mitochondria are being affected, then the amount of melatonin is also being affected. This is another way your liver, its mitochondria and melatonin are negatively affected, this situation caused from your intestinal microbiota.

Multiple studies have shown people with cirrhosis have bacterial strains in their intestines not found in those without cirrhosis. Also, people with cirrhosis have many different types of bacterial strains, upwards of 30-40 types of bacteria which is not seen in those without cirrhosis. The cause of the cirrhosis is the pathogenic bacteria trans-locating through the hepatic portal vein, thereby affecting the liver and mitochondria.

Here is another fascinating fact regarding the gut microbiota affecting the liver, and it still reads like Sci-Fi even though this information is decades old - studies show that unhealthy types of bacteria in the gut alter liver function. One such study from 1960 showed a difference in bilirubin metabolism in germ-free rats compared to bilirubin metabolism in those same rats after they had fecal transplants from conventional rats.[211] This difference in bilirubin metabolism could only have been due to the introduction of the bacteria as that was the only factor that changed. In a 1977 study the researchers saw there was a difference in bile acid elimination between germ-free rats compared to conventional rats.[212] This is important because currently we know that a change in bile acids changes several metabolic pathways influencing glucose metabolism, fat metabolism, cholesterol metabolism, and enzymes for detoxification functions. A study from 1969 also found those same results and in the same study these researchers also determined that there is a difference in the excretion of steroid hormones in germ-free rats compared to conventional rats.[213]

Another crucial consequence of intestinal bacterial overgrowth is the common toxin the bacteria give off, known as lipopolysaccharides. This toxin also trans-locates from the intestinal tract to the liver and it is known to cause liver damage and damage to other parts of your body. (Some sources use the term "endotoxin, which is the same thing.) It is known that lipopolysaccharides/endotoxins cause changes to the immune system, lymph system, brain chemistry, kidneys, heart, the arteries and veins, reproductive hormones, and the liver. It is also well known that lipopolysaccharides contribute significantly to the progression of septic shock.

A significant research study by Seki and colleagues proved that the intestinal bacteria/microflora was the main source of lipopolysaccharides entering the liver through the hepatic portal vein. This proved to be "an important prerequisite for the development of liver fibrosis during chronic liver injury."[214] This research is very important in showing how your liver health and your gut microbiota are integrally related.

Another significant article is in the *British Journal of Pharmacology*, titled "The multiple organ dysfunction syndrome caused by endotoxin in the rat: attenuation of liver dysfunction by inhibitors of nitric oxide synthase."[215] In this study, researchers found that lipopolysaccharides "caused a profound hypotension associated with decreases in cardiac output and oxygen delivery, lactic acidosis, renal and liver dysfunction, and thrombocytopenia."[216] This means that the lipopolysaccharides caused a heart rate so low that it resulted in extremely low blood pressure, that does not deliver enough oxygen to the entire body and results in lactic acid build up, negatively affecting the kidneys and liver and causing low platelets, resulting in a lack of clotting. Their study revealed how multiple organs are affected by lipopolysaccharides.

Liver cirrhosis is a disease that is prevalent worldwide and mostly preventable. It is the result of a combination of chronic liver diseases and/or chronic health problems in a different organ which then secondarily affect the liver. An example is pathogenic bacteria from the gut and the lipopolysaccharides from those bacteria trans-locating to the liver and then negatively affecting the mitochondria in the liver. Cirrhosis happens over several years. Liver cirrhosis occurs because the cells of the liver die as a consequence of defective and decreased mitochondria. (There are several cascades that occur as a result of diminishing mitochondrial numbers, this is the simplistic version.) Cirrhosis will cause death unless the person gets a liver transplant. When mitochondria become defective or lessened in numbers, there is an increase of ROS as these two factors have an inverse relationship. This scenario is seen in numerous diseases that impact the liver. Due to the failing status of the liver unable to perform its necessary jobs - the entire body gets affected.

Examples of diseases that affect the liver and then subsequently other organs are metabolic syndrome, type 2 diabetes, hepatitis B and C, alcoholism, fatty liver disease and non-alcoholic fatty liver, and liver cancer. Because it takes years for cirrhosis to develop, and glaring symptoms don't manifest until the problem is drastic, most people do not even realize they might be heading that way.

Let's take a look at some study results on the liver and gut and the inter-relationship these 2 organs have on each other. These researchers were looking at the relationship of the gut microbiota in patients with Hepatitis C virus infection, or HCV: "The impact of HCV infection on intestinal permeability allows gut disbiosis starting, maintenance and its proinflammatory effect until liver cirrhosis and HCC (hepatocellular carcinoma) development. HCV eradication has unraveled the strong impact of gut microbiota unbalance on liver disease development"[217]

Another study concluded that non-alcoholic fatty liver

disease, or NAFLD, occurs as a result of the gut microbiota through a multi-step complicated process that impacts liver metabolism, metabolites, and choline. "Such significant association indicates that the altered gut-microbial metabolism of choline plays a role in the development of NAFLD."[218] These researchers concluded: "Our observations indicate that gut-microbial metabolism alters the metabolism of the mammalian host."[219]

Another group of researchers saw cause-and-effect disease processes in the liver as a result of damaged or low levels of mitochondria. As a consequence of decreased mitochondrial activity, the rise in "ROS produced in mitochondria may be the main cause of nuclear-gene mutation in carcinogenesis. The mitochondrial dysfunction and overproduction of ROS plays a key role in progression of chronic hepatitis C and ethanol-induced liver injury. Ethanol also causes bacterial translocation in the intestine and the resulting lipopolysaccharides (LPS) activates Kupffer cells to produce pro-inflammatory cytokines."[220] They stated they suspected the increase in ROS, or reactive oxygen species, causes non-alcoholic steatohepatitis, which is non-alcoholic fatty liver disease that also has inflammation in the liver and liver cell damage along with the fat stored in the liver. From the information in this study you can see how a problem in the liver will lead to a number of other chronic health problems.

An important factor to consider is how the liver gets affected in metabolic syndrome, and type 2 diabetes. As the liver plays a major role in our energy/glucose homeostasis, diseases that manifest in low or high blood glucose levels have a negative effect to the liver and specifically the mitochondria of the liver. The mitochondria get changed structurally and functionally from low or high blood glucose levels, which leads to an increase in reactive oxygen species, or ROS, which are free radicals. And this is where the scales start to tip, once the mitochondria in the liver cannot perform their job, ROS continue to increase. That increase in ROS becomes more and more of a burden on the mitochondria, crippling them in an escalating manner.

A diet high in processed foods is taxing to the liver because of the man-made chemicals present, all requiring enzymes in the mitochondria to reduce them to a form that can then get eliminated. You read earlier how processed foods create a gut microbiota that is dominated by disease-causing organisms, which is Step 1. Step 2 in this cascade is the man-made chemicals in processed foods being delivered to the liver to be broken down. That is the job of the mitochondria in the liver, which are very capable. If this was just a rare occurrence it would not be a problem, the liver can do it. However, think about what a heavy load is placed on the liver to constantly break down man-made chemicals in a person with a high consumption of processed foods over the course of years. Step 3 in this process occurs when the bacteria in the gut begins to migrate to the liver. Step 4 is the effect to the liver from the lipopolysaccharides from the pathogenic bacteria. Think about the cumulative effect over years. Now add in the fact that more than half of adult Americans take prescription and/or over-the-counter medications daily. Combine all these individual steps together and you can see the demand on the liver over the years will have an effect.

Sugar is another problem for the liver. The details of sugar consumption in America are discussed in the upcoming section "Sugar Reality," but here we will discuss how sugar affects the liver.

Since 1980 there has been a steady rise in non-alcoholic fatty liver disease, or NAFLD, and non-alcoholic steatohepatitis, NASH, and this climb is parallel with the increases in obesity, type 2 diabetes, and metabolic syndrome. All of these curves on a graph run parallel to the curve representing America's increase in sugar consumption. By 2011 NASH was the third leading cause for liver transplants[221] and is projected to be the leading cause for liver transplants by 2020.[222] It is a fact that the Western diet most commonly eaten here in the United States causes an increase in body weight, the weight of the liver, inflammatory markers, cholesterol, triglycerides, and glucose levels.[223] All these factors impact liver health, and sugar is a driving factor for each.

When you eat sugar in excess of what your body needs to function daily, the excess gets stored in fat in the liver as well as in muscles. Fructose, or fruit sugar, functions a little differently as it gets moved directly from the small intestines to your liver to be processed. Then your liver decides whether to release it as glucose or store it as fat. Much of the added sugars in foods in America are a combination of glucose and fructose, placing a large burden on your liver. This is why Americans are developing fatty livers, which is why there is the parallel in curves for sugar consumption and rates of NAFLD and NASH.

It is possible to keep your liver healthy through lifestyle choices. Keeping your liver healthy will impart a dramatic consequence to your overall health, your brain, and how you age. By mitigating the burden of oxidation, free radicals, you will increase not only your longevity but also your quality of life. If you have a lifestyle that will support the health of your mitochondria, you will increase your longevity and have a positive effect to your quality of life.

Everything Old Is New Again

The more research that is done on the microbiome, the more it is pointing to a fact that has been completely understood and utilized for centuries by Acupuncturists and Herbalists, and that is the knowledge that the human body is a Whole. The parts cannot be separated out in order to take care of one disease.

Currently modern medicine has grouped together diseases that even 20 years ago were not seen as related from the Western Medicine standpoint. The term to describe this is "pathogenetic commonalities." Pathogenetic commonalities looks at the spectrum of one disease and connects its propensity to developing one or more diseases due to shared pathological processes and disease progression. Here are some examples of pathogenetic commonalities.

A person with rheumatoid arthritis has a higher chance of having a heart attack and gout. A person with one autoimmune condition has a higher chance of developing two more autoimmune disorders. These are all on a spectrum and are results of how long that person's body has dealt with systemic inflammation and has had to accommodate problems in the body. Once a second or third disease sets in, it shows you progression of disease affecting more tissues. Once someone has diabetes, they have a higher chance of having a stroke, heart attack, hypertension, and high cholesterol. This propensity towards these other health problems is toward all of them, not just a higher risk of getting one of them, it is all of them. Let's back up from diabetes for one moment to look at metabolic syndrome. People with metabolic syndrome are headed toward type 2 diabetes; once they progress to diabetes, their risk of those same pathogenetic commonalities is present. The last group of pathogenic commonalities being brought up here is what you read about earlier in this book, people with digestive disorders commonly end up having Alzheimer's or Parkinson's disease.

While the term "pathogenetic commonalities" is newly coined, it has always been the perspective of those of us in the Wholistic field. We look at the whole and see what tissues, organs, or glands are not functioning properly and see the downstream and upstream effects. The Wholistic practitioner then treats the manifestation along with the problem coming from upstream that is driving the symptoms, thereby treating the whole person. We do this because that is what the whole human body is, an organism, made up of 12 major organs and nine major glands, that take part in 10 systems, which all need to work together systematically and harmoniously in order to be healthy. When one organ, gland, or system is malfunctioning, it leads to other malfunctions. Even one organ not functioning well affects the other organs, glands, and systems. It is a matter of how long that one organ or gland can hobble along with a decreased ability to do its job, resulting in an increasing burden impacting other organs, glands, and systems, in a domino effect.

Vital Factors for Your Health

The next two sections contain some important information on other factors that play a vital role to your health. There is some information about each of these factors here, but it is not a comprehensive report. There is considerable research on each topic and while these factors do play a role in health, and disease, they are part of the equation and not the entire focus of this book. The information presented on these topics is valuable for your health and for the people you love.

Sugar Reality

The rate of sugar consumption has steadily risen since the 1800s. The earliest record of sugar consumption in America shows that in 1822 the average American consumed about 7 grams of sugar each day, or about 1½ teaspoons. Currently, the average 12-ounce soda contains 35 grams of sugar, or 9 teaspoons of sugar, translating to 135 calories. Other sugar-sweetened beverages, juices, lemonades, sports drinks, etc., average 25 grams of sugar in just 8 ounces, which is about 6 teaspoons of sugar. Put another way, in 1822 the average American would have drank that 12-ounce soda over the course of 5 days! And that would be it for their sugar intake! Do you know anybody that would drink one 12-ounce can of soda in the span of five days and *not* have any other sugary foods over those 5 days?! I think not! And Americans are in for more sugar. Read on to see how much sugar was projected to be imported and produced in America in 2019!

In 1822 the average American consumed about 7 pounds of sugar each year. By 1880 that number rose to about 30 pounds per person per year. By 1940 that number grew to 80 pounds of sugar each year per person until World War II, after which consumption decreased for just a few years before steadily rising again. In 1990 sugar consumption increased to 100 pounds per person per year! By 2000 it rose to about 107 pounds for each person every year. In 2017, the average American consumed an estimated 117 pounds of sugar every year. Keep in mind that is averaged out, but there are many people who purposely do not consume much sugar which means that there are millions of people consuming even more than 117 pounds of sugar each year. When compared to 7 pounds per person in 1822 sugar consumption per person per year rose by 110 pounds! "Can I get an OMG!"

Researchers looking at the 1999-2006 National Health and Nutrition Examination Survey, NHANES, noted that adults were getting about 1/6, about 15.8%, of their calories every day from added sugars.[224] This was a "substantial increase from 1977-1978, when added sugars contributed only 10.6%" of the daily calories.[225] The 2011-2014 NHANES reported that the average daily intake of sugar-sweetened beverages for Americans daily was 6.5% of their daily calories.[226] On the US Department of Agriculture website in an article from 2012 it states that the average American is eating or drinking 34 teaspoons of sugar each day which amounts to at least 500 calories.[227]

Currently the American Heart Association is recommending that Americans reduce their daily sugar intake by two-thirds, from the current average of 34 teaspoons of sugar daily to the upper limit of 10 teaspoons for women and 15 for men. But, you don't have to stop there. There is no need for sugar consumption, not even 2 teaspoons per day. You can cut sugar completely from your diet and the consequences would be a dramatic increase in your health.

Just one more look at some numbers as relates to sugar, because it is eye opening. Following are some numbers from the United States Department of Agriculture Foreign Agricultural Service on sugar production and consumption through the years. For each year listed, this is the total sugar listed for human consumption. These are the combined totals of beet sugar, cane sugar, and imported sugar for human consumption in the United States for each year:

Year 1995: 18,674,000 pounds[228]
Year 2000: 19,954,000 pounds[229]
Year 2005: 20,086,000 pounds[230]
Year 2010: 21,984,000 pounds[231]
Year 2015: 23,866,000 pounds[232]
Year 2018: 24,132,000 pounds[233]

In the span of just 23 years the sugar consumption for

just the United States increased 5,458,000 pounds. It increased by almost a third! In just 23 years!

This is the most sugar Americans have ever consumed. The agriculture industry is producing it because there is a demand for it. If you look at your diet, can you see foods that you are eating that have sugar in them? What about the foods you feed your family? Do your habits and the habits of your family help drive the demand for increased sugar production? If you answered yes, now think about how sick do you want to be? How sick do you want your family to be?

It is important to see the escalating amounts of sugar that have been produced because it is part of the equation in the health crisis in America today. Literally, tons of sugar are being produced, the food industry will use that ever-increasing amount in the foods being eaten, and we Americans will continue to experience escalating, and preventable, health problems.

Here is more data from the United States Department of Agriculture for the same years as shown above, showing that while the United States is consuming more sugar, it is exporting less.

In 1995: exported 1,036,000 pounds and consumed 18,674,000 pounds.[234] In 2000: exported 218,000 pounds and consumed 19,954,000 pounds.[235] In 2005: exported 486,000 pounds and consumed 20,408,6000 pounds.[236] In 2010: exported 458,000 pounds and consumed 21,984,000 pounds.[237] In 2015: exported 346,000 pounds and consumed 23,866,000 pounds.[238] In 2018: exported 302,000 pounds and consumed 24,132,000 pounds.[239]

The health problems related to sugar consumption are numerous. In fact, I believe that sugar consumption can be related to most health problems, as sugar causes inflammation, and chronic systemic inflammation contributes to every disease state by altering the body's terrain/microbiome. Chronic inflammation is an altered environment that affects your arteries, organs, nerves, brain, joints, muscles, and all organs. Chronic inflammation keeps your immune system on heightened alert, which can then cause over-reactions from the immune system that are autoimmune problems. In most cases this cascade of events begins in the intestinal tract and takes years before progressing to autoimmune problems.

Now let's look at the enormously popular drinks that Americans consume daily, aka "liquid sugar." Sugar-sweetened beverages have been in existence since the 1600s while carbonated sugar-sweetened drinks have been peddled since the 1700s. Sugar-sweetened drinks grew in mass popularity as a consequence of a few factors, with technology playing a starring role. The ability to mass produce sugar so that it became more available only became possible as a result of technology.

Technology was also the conduit for mass production of bottles, caps, and lids. And of course, technology also played a necessary role in the filling of the bottles en masse which was required in order for sugar-sweetened drinks to grow to the level of availability we see today. Even the explosion of fruit juice for young kids is directly tied to advances in packaging. Picture the little aluminum juice pouches that every parent feels safe handing one over to their toddler. It's not glass, so if their little hands drop it, it will just bounce.

The NHANES survey of 2011-2014 showed that 53.6% of American male adults 20 years old and above drank at least one sugar-sweetened beverage each day and 45.1% of American female adults 20 years old and above drank at least one sugar-sweetened beverage every day.[240] Over the course of a year, by just eliminating sugar-sweetened beverages a person would make a difference to their weight and their overall health. It has been shown that by "drinking just one 20-ounce bottle of a sugary beverage per day can result in gaining 25 extra pounds per year."[241]

The results from the NHANES ending in 2014 showed not just the health problems that are often seen in people drinking sugar sweetened beverages but also showed a trend in early deaths as a result of that consumption.[242] The results also showed increased early death for women even if those drinks were artificially sweetened. [243] The positive association of early deaths among women due to sugar-sweetened beverages and artificially sweetened beverages was for all-cause mortality and cardiovascular disease.[244] For men, the results showed an increase in early death from all-cause mortality and cardiovascular disease from sugar sweetened beverages; men consuming artificially sweetened beverages did not show an increase in cardiovascular disease.[245] This study's report is valuable information that all Americans should know as it can change life expectancy and quality of life, whether it is cardiovascular disease or another chronic health problem. Serious chronic health problems do alter the quality of life. So even before a disease causes death, it has dramatically affected a person's life, usually making the last several years of that person's life miserable and filled with suffering. Included in this scenario are numerous doctors' visits, money for medications, and most likely medical procedures.

In the latest data available from the NHANES of 2011-2014, sweetened beverages were being consumed at a rate of 49.3% on any given day by Americans.[246] Men usually consume more SSB (sugar-sweetened beverages) than women. 53.6% of men consume an SSB on any given day while 45.1% of women will consume an SSB on any given day.[247] Men consume an average 179 calories from SSB on a daily basis, contributing 6.9% of their total daily calories.[248] Women consumed an average 113 calories from SSB, contributing 6.1% of total calories for the day.[249]

In 2010 the *American Journal of Clinical Nutrition* reported on a study showing cardiometabolic health problems in the people drinking higher amounts of sugar-sweetened beverages.[250] ("Cardiometabolic" is problems with insulin resistance, impaired glucose tolerance, increased fat levels in the blood, increased intra-abdominal fat tissue, heart disease, hypertension, and stroke.) This article was based on the CARDIA study, an amazing study that yielded numerous informative results that thus far has resulted in over 770 papers and has been the catalyst for several research studies to further our understanding on diet and its effects to health.[251] Also in 2010, a group of researchers performed a cross-sectional study from data in the National Health and Nutrition Examination Survey 1999-2006. These researchers saw a direct and "significant" response in the blood lipid levels of adults in relation to how much added sugar was in their diet.[252] This occurs because when blood sugar/glucose levels are high, the compensatory/protective mechanism in the body to reduce that high glucose level is to shuffle that excess glucose into triglycerides, a form of fat carried in the blood throughout your body. Increased triglycerides are an indicator of other conditions that increase the risk of heart disease.

A very important paper that was published in November 2016 in the *Journal of the American Medical Association* should be read by all Americans. This paper resourced documents from 1965 from the Sugar Research Foundation, in which the authors revealed how the Sugar Research Foundation manipulated research about sugar's role in coronary heart disease.[253] The Sugar Research Foundation shifted the blame for increases in coronary heart disease to fats. Think about it, even now in 2021 we usually think about fats as playing a role in coronary heart disease without a thought about sugar as a contributing factor.[254] In 1965 the Sugar Research Foundation used the articles its authors wrote to shape public policy regarding sugar consumption for decades to come.[255] Of course the result was the sugar industry was able to increase profits for sugar producers.[256] This paper opened my eyes. We all need to be wary of "research," as in knowing who the authors are, who is paying them, and what the motivation is. Fortunately now researchers do disclose this information.

The authors of the 2016 paper did not stop there. Their next paper on this topic was published in *PLoSBiology* in November 2017. It looked at another study that had important information about sugar consumption and health and what happened to that research, which just happened to be sponsored by the Sugar Research Foundation. This 2017 research paper is based on internal Sugar Research Foundation documents from a research project from 1967-1971 funded by the Sugar Research Foundation. The 1967 research project was actually discontinued and its results never published once the researchers discovered that sucrose changed the bladder environment altering the presence of enzymes that then leads to bladder cancer.[257]

Following that result, the lead researcher then informed the Vice President of Research for the Sugar Research Foundation that a high sucrose diet led to increased levels of triglycerides.[258] Not only did the Sugar Research Foundation stop the research project and not publish any of the results, they actually hid those results.[259] (If this sounds familiar, it's exactly what the tobacco industry did with its knowledge from the mid-1940s that smoking caused increases in lung cancer. And it's also what happened recently with opioids and information as to how addictive they are, which was known.)

Your health will determine how you will age. Aging comes down to the health of your gut microbiota. The longer a person has inflammatory intestinal problems the faster it will lead to an unhealthy/altered microbiota of each organ, leading faster to diseases. Pathogenic bacteria, chronic systemic inflammation, and ROS cause aging to your cells, organs, glands, and brain. This fascinating study on the people living in Goatian village in the Hunan province in China proved how important the gut microbiota is to longevity. The people in Goatian live an average of 92 years, while the general lifespan for people in China is 74.83 years. Also of note is that the people from Goatian do not have chronic diseases. The gut microbiota of the elder people ranging from 50 to over 90 years old was analyzed and "revealed much greater species diversity than that observed in the control group (healthy subjects from other areas in China, average age of 50 years)."[260]

The Other Vital Factor: Calorie Consumption

While the huge increases in sugar consumption are definitely a factor in the health crisis in America, there is another factor that has to be accounted for. That other factor is over-all food, or calorie, consumption. Americans are eating more food than they need. Numerous studies and graphs showing different types of foods being consumed all show an increase in food consumption of all types. We are consuming more vegetables, fruits, sugar, proteins, starches, and fats than our bodies need to function. Any extra calories consumed that the body doesn't need to utilize goes into storage, meaning they get stored as fat.

Vary Your Foods

It is very important to vary your foods. Most people in the industrial world eat the same five to seven foods on a repeated weekly, if not daily, basis. These same foods are the preferred tastes for each person. Those same foods offer the same phytonutrients repeatedly, meaning your body is not getting other phytonutrients that it needs.

The other problem with eating the same foods repeatedly is that it results in a limited range of bacteria in the intestinal tract, whereas our intestinal tract should be home to over 1,000 healthy types of bacteria that assist in breaking down our foods and waste. Remember, our gut microbiota is created through supply and demand - the supply provided into the gut causes that specific demand for those foods to get broken down. This results in organisms that are capable of breaking down the foods eaten. If a limited range of foods is eaten repeatedly, it will result in just the types of microbes that are breaking down those repeated foods. As stated earlier, people with IBS and IBD have a limited variety of organisms in the gut compared with people who do not have either of those intestinal disorders.

"The taxonomic diversity of the fecal microbiota of individuals on habitual Western diets appears to be less than for those consuming plant-based diets. Also, individuals who are obese or have type 2 diabetes, inflammatory diseases (osteoarthritis) and other major health problems (prevalent in Western societies) have a sub-optimal fecal microbiota profile."[261] To be very specific, the fecal microbiota profile has less diversity compared to healthy controls.[262] [263]

In 2012 this study found "The fecal hydrogenotrophic microbiota of native Africans, whose diet is low in animal products, compared to that of African Americans and European Americans consuming a typical Western diet was more diverse and contained different populations of hydrogenotrophic *Archaea* and methanogenic *Archaea* as well as Sulfate Reducing Bacteria populations."[264] The researchers saw that the Native Africans compared to the African Americans and European Americans "harbored the full range of targeted hydrogenotrophic groups."[265] The Native African diet is high in resistant starches, plants, and very low in animal protein. Their high resistant starch intake drives a "greater microbial fermentation"[266] and results in low levels of sulfate-reducing bacteria which is seen in higher amounts in the African Americans and European Americans in this study. "The differences in bacterial community structures of Native African populations were reflective of the diets of the hosts. Those on Western diets, characterized by higher intakes of dietary animal proteins (meat, milk, and eggs), may deliver greater amounts of sulphur compounds to the colonic microbiota"[267] This matters because sulfate-reducing bacteria "has been linked with chronic inflammatory disorders of the colon."[268] And the Native Africans had low levels of sulfate-reducing bacteria and have low rates of inflammatory bowel diseases.

Phytonutrients - What Are They?

You will hear more and more talk about phytonutrients and why they matter for your health. Phytonutrients are the compounds in vegetables, fruits, nuts, seeds, beans, and legumes – basically compounds from plants - that provide the health benefits our bodies need. The word "Phytonutrient" derives from the Greek word "Phyto" for plants and the word "nutrients." You can think of plants as thee strongest-most-potent-completely-natural-mega-vitamin that could ever be made! Plants all have an enormous amount of diverse bioactive substances that are incredibly beneficial for our bodies and brain.

These phytonutrients develop in plants as their defense against bacteria, fungi, viruses, the sun, the cold, and even diseases. All organisms have a will to survive and need a defense system, as without a defense system no species - plant, animal, or human - will survive. As an Herbalist, I have been explaining this for decades to my patients: an herb used for medicinal purposes confers the protective mechanisms it has for itself. These mechanisms/phytonutrients allow that plant to defend itself against organisms or the environment, which is how the plant continues to exist.

As scientific research progresses, we know more about the science and chemical components of plants than any other time in history. It is enthralling knowing the molecular structures and the clarity of the details in the phytonutrient categories, thanks to all the research scientists. They have dedicated their lives to informing us about the vital information we need to make the best choices in taking care of ourselves. I truly find all the information available to us valuable as information serves the purpose of educating us so we can make better choices. An important fact, and this is not in any way to take away from the research and the dedicated scientists performing these studies because their research is valuable to all people not just professionals in the health field, every culture, going back thousands of years, has used plants to their advantage for health purposes before knowing about their molecular structure, and some still do to this day. These cultures saw the results of what the plants did and still do.

For decades we have all known that for good health we needed to get calcium, potassium, Vitamin A, the B Vitamins, Vitamin C, Vitamin D, Vitamin K, as well as other minerals. But now we know that our cells need a range of phytonutrients. Phytonutrients cause biochemical events in our bodies that we need in order to be healthy. As we have seen, it is the organisms in the gut microbiota that are needed to extract these phytonutrients. And fascinatingly, these phytonutrients directly alter which organisms will make up the gut microbiota.

Phytonutrients encompass a few different classes, some

of which may be familiar, some not. Familiar groups include carotenoids, flavonoids, polyphenols, indoles, lignans, and isoflavones. Each group conveys distinct health benefits when we eat them. Following is some basic information on some of the groups and why they matter to your health.

This section introduces the phytonutrients and how they benefit us. The next section, "The Rainbow of Phytonutrients," breaks down the different phytonutrients in vegetables by color and lists which foods contain those phytonutrients.

Carotenoids: Carotenoids are crucial for cell-to-cell-communication. They are found in yellow, orange, red, and green vegetables, which get their coloring from the carotenoids. You may already know you will get vitamin A when you eat carrots, bell peppers, and other foods with carotenoids, this is because carotenoids are pro-vitamin A. The pro-vitamin A carotenoids that get converted to vitamin A in our bodies are alpha- carotene, beta-carotene, and beta-cryptoxanthin. There are over 600 known carotenoids, and though less than 50 of these are pro-vitamin A, some of the others are known to confer health benefits as well. Getting optimum carotenoids will provide you with the levels of vitamin A that is necessary for proper growth and development, cell differentiation, vision, a healthy immune system, and reproduction. Vitamin A is used by your lungs, kidneys, and heart.

Some of the other beneficial carotenoids are lycopene, lutein, and zeaxanthin. Lycopene reduces DNA damage from free radicals, reduces platelets from clumping together, reduces cytokines that contribute to inflammation, helps fat metabolism, reduces C-reactive protein, and reduces blood pressure. Lutein and zeaxanthin are usually found together in plants and are crucial for the development of the eyes in utero and necessary throughout life to keep vision healthy. Many studies have proven that lutein and zeaxanthin do make a difference as we go through life by helping you to avoid age-related eye diseases, such as cataracts and age-related macular degeneration.

Glucosinolates are present in cruciferous vegetables and through the process of metabolism they get altered and become indoles, thiocyanates, isothiocyanates, and nitriles, to name a few of the substances they become. The glucosinolates are found in pungent plants like broccoli, bok choy, cabbage, kale, Brussels sprouts, and horseradish. (A comprehensive list of cruciferous vegetables is in the following section "The Rainbow of Phytonutrients.") These glucosinolates are the catalysts that stimulate your liver to produce antioxidants to scavenge free radicals, thereby curtailing damage to DNA. Cruciferous vegetables are commonly thought of as anti-cancer, and most of the anti-cancer abilities of deep green vegetables are attributed to these indoles and isothiocyanates from the glucosinolates.

Another absolutely alluring fact regarding indoles is the protection they confer to the cells of the intestinal tract. A study found that indoles maintain the health of the intestinal barrier by increasing the ability of the barrier to resist pathogenic E. coli and by reducing the inflammatory response that pathogenic E. coli sets off, which propagates its ability to colonize.[269] It was also discovered that high levels of indoles reduced the ability of pathogenic Salmonella and E. coli to create a biofilm[270], which is a protective shield that bacteria build around themselves in which they reproduce while also reducing their chances of coming under attack by healthy bacteria or anti-biotics, think if it as a force-field of sorts. These facts alone should convince you to keep your indole intake high.

Polyphenols are a huge class of phytonutrients, with over 8,000 different phenols. Each phenol has a distinct molecular structure and, as a result, could perform distinctive functions in our body, which is determined by the individual molecular structure. All of the polyphenols have strong antioxidant effects for our bodies. Each group of polyphenols confers different effects in our bodies. You will read more about the individual groups and how they make a difference in our bodies in the following section, "Rainbow of Phytonutrients." Within the class of polyphenols are a number of other families of substances. The largest class is the family of flavonoids/bioflavonoids, which itself has several sub-classes.

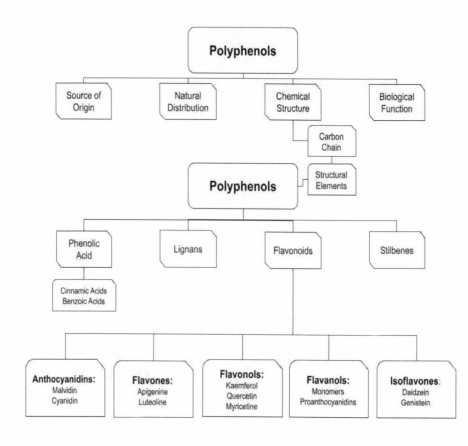

Flavonoids encompass anthocyanins, flavanoles, flavonols, flavanones, isoflavones, chalcones, lignans, among others. Flavonoids have proven to have anti-viral[271], antibacterial[272], and anti-fungal effects[273]; reduce inflammation[274]; cause cell-death in malignant cells[275] (cell death is a programmed component in cells and necessary when cells become old and are not functioning correctly); and inhibit inflammatory mediators like Cox-2 and cytokines among others[276]. Flavonoids have numerous health benefits and are even associated with a reduced risk of several different types of cancers[277].

Isoflavones are a subset of flavonoids. For three decades there has been tremendous interest and research into the isoflavone from soy products. This interest was driven by the lower rates of breast and prostate cancer in Asia, where there is high soy intake. Today, higher intake of soy, or isoflavones, is still being studied as a means of reducing the risk of breast and prostate cancer. One group of researchers determined that 10mg of isoflavone intake every day can reduce a young woman's chance of having breast cancer.[278]

There are other immensely helpful benefits from eating isoflavones. It has been observed in multiple studies that a higher intake of soy and isoflavones lowers your risk of having coronary heart disease.[279] Some of this is attributed to the fact that soy isoflavones lower LDL cholesterol levels and triglycerides, while also increasing the HDL levels.[280] It has been frequently reported that isoflavones have an anti-diabetic effect and can help in managing the complications from diabetes.[281] [282] Some of the complications often seen in people with diabetes is the development of coronary heart disease, high levels of LDL cholesterol, and triglycerides – all conditions that soy isoflavones have been proven to help.

Another benefit of soy isoflavones is to the liver, as they are shown to help with alcoholic fatty liver disease and non-alcoholic fatty liver disease, decreasing the fibrosis of liver cells.[283] This same author also noted that other isoflavones also help reduce fatty acid formation.[284]

Soy isoflavones are known to contribute antioxidant help

to the body, which has positive ramifications throughout the body. The strong antioxidant effects from soy isoflavones contribute to helping the liver by assisting the detoxifying liver enzymes in their job. And it is thought that the antioxidant effects also make a difference to the brain as soy isoflavones have been seen to prevent cognitive impairment[285] [286] and have a neuroprotective effect.[287] It is also through the antioxidant activity that soy isoflavones help reduce the risk of cancer.

Soy contains the highest amount of isoflavones, but other foods have isoflavones too. Here are some good ways to get isoflavones without having soy: pinto beans, kidney beans, navy beans, chickpeas, split peas, mung beans, cannellini beans, fava beans, walnuts, peanuts, pistachios, and sunflower seeds. As you can see from this list, isoflavones are present in foods of several different colors which is why this list of the foods was placed here as opposed to the following section, "The Rainbow of Phytonutrients", which contains lists of the phytonutrients in foods in specific color ranges. It is known that the isoflavones in chickpeas are a very good substitute for soy isoflavones.[288]

One more polyphenol that must be discussed is quercetin. Quercetin is in every fruit, vegetable, and grain. How incredibly beneficial quercetin is for your health cannot be stressed enough. Scientific studies reveal that quercetin helps your body in these ways:

❖ Reduces inflammation by stopping inflammatory proteins.[289] [290] [291]

❖ Protects brain health reducing risk from neurodegeneration.[292] [293] [294]
❖ Strong antioxidant effects that increase overall health, reducing risk from all disease processes.[295] [296] [297] [298]
❖ Reduces blood pressure.[299] [300] [301]
❖ Helpful in preventing heart conditions.[302] [303] [304]
❖ Reduces risk of cancer and there are studies discussing using quercetin to treat cancer.[305] [306] [307]

There are thousands of studies on the effects of quercetin, and for each benefit listed above there are many more studies.

Here is a title from a scientific study that should catch your attention, "The Flavinoids Quercetin, Kaempferol, and Myricetin Inhibit Hepatocyte Growth Factor-Induced Medulloblastoma Cell Migration"[308], the researchers of this study saw that plant phytonutrients blocked a necessary pathway in medulloblastoma, a brain cancer in children, and also blocked metastasis.[309] It was observed that the amounts of those phytonutrients that had that effect in blocking the necessary pathway was at a level that can be achieved just by eating the plant foods, no supplementation necessary.[310] The World Cancer Research Fund International in 2018 stated, "Overall the evidence is more persuasive of a protective effect and that greater consumption of non-starchy vegetables and or fruit helps protect against a number of aerodigestive cancers and some other cancers."[311]

Through laboratory studies, the National Cancer Institute has seen that there are more than 1,000 phytonutrients that have the ability to prevent cancer activity. Also, in each serving of vegetables there could be 100 different phytonutrients.[312]

The Rainbow of Phytonutrients

This section presents a breakdown of the different phytonutrients in vegetables by color. (Fruits of the same color also provide those same phytonutrients, but I always emphasize eating more vegetables than fruit.) A general rule of thumb: the deeper the color the more of those specific phytonutrients that vegetable has to offer. As an example, the deeper green vegetables provide much more phytonutrients than the lighter green vegetables. With that being said, there are white vegetables that are very good for you, and should be part of your regular diet.

White vegetables are high in allyl sulfides, allicin, which have been shown to lower cholesterol and reduce the risk of stomach and colon cancer. The other phytonutrients in white vegetables are EGCG, which is a family of five catechins: epicatechin, gallocatechin, epigallocatechin, epicatechin gallate, and epigallocatechin gallate. EGCG has been studied a lot for its numerous benefits; it is strongly anti-inflammatory and an extremely good antioxidant. Several studies have looked at the neuroprotective abilities of EGCG, mostly from green tea, but white vegetables contain a good dose of EGCG. The strong antioxidant ability is thought to be how EGCG is able to protect the brain. There have been some results showing EGCG helps combat metabolic syndrome and diabetes by making cells more sensitive to insulin.

Anthocyanidins are another phytonutrient in white vegetables. These are in the same family as anthocyanins, which are found in red vegetables. The difference between these two closely named phytonutrients is the detail of sugar. Anthocyanidins in white vegetables are not bound with a sugar molecule whereas anthocyanins in red vegetables are coupled with a sugar molecule. Most of the research studies are on anthocyanins, but they do apply to the anthocyanidins since they are same minus the sugar. In fact there is even more value to the anthocyanidins as studies have shown that anthocyanidins have a higher ORAC value than anthocyanins, ORAC is the Oxygen Radical Absorbance Capacity. The higher the ORAC value the higher the antioxidant effect from that food.

Anthocyanidins in white vegetables are a powerhouse phytonutrient and a very powerful antioxidant. There are more than 635 anthocyanins in nature.[313] These powerful antioxidants are so potent that they are capable of reducing the chances of obesity, reducing secondary health problems in diabetes, helpful in preventing cardiovascular disease, and are especially helpful in lowering the risk of cancers.[314] Something to keep in mind here is the pathogenetic commonality of these disease processes - obesity increases the risk for developing type 2 diabetes which increases the risk of developing cardiovascular disease; and obesity is also a pathogenetic commonality for several cancers. Eating lots of white vegetables can reduce your risk of all of these. Anthocyanins reduce inflammation and blood pressure and promote blood vessel health – this is mostly due to the powerful antioxidant function combined with the anti-inflammatory abilities as this combination directly helps the blood vessels by lowering the pressure. It has been observed that anthocyanins help protect against blood clotting. Anthocyanins play a role in protecting cells as well. A few studies have shown that some anthocyanins can cross the blood-brain barrier, thereby playing a role in neuroprotection.[315] [316] The anthocyanins that cross the blood brain barrier have a positive effect to a few of the neurotransmitters and actively influence some biochemical signaling.[317] [318] Anthocyanins have also been shown in scientific studies to have anti-viral abilities, promote liver health by protecting the liver, and help visual health.

Isothiocyanate and quercetin are also present in white vegetables. These phyotnutrients are found in other vegetables and have each been the focus of many research studies. Most of the studies have used green vegetables to see the impact from isothiocyanate, red and purple vegetables to see the benefits from anthocyanins, which is why these phytonutrients are discussed in more detail in those color categories. Quercetin was discussed in the previous section, and as stated earlier, quercetin is in all vegetable and fruits including the white vegetables. This is unique as all the other phytonutrients are associated with colors, but quercetin exists in a range of colors in vegetables and fruit and is present in the cruciferous family, which contains several white vegetables.

Studies have shown that some of the phytonutrients in white vegetables have anti-cancer properties, particularly against colon and breast cancer. Related to lowering the risk for breast cancer is the hormonal balance that white vegetables convey. The phytonutrients in white vegetables help strengthen your immune system. Also very important is the strong anti-inflammatory properties in white vegetables coupled with the other phytonutrients that conveys to people who regularly eat white vegetables and fruit a reduced risk of stroke[319] according to some researchers. The researchers in this study discovered that it was the white vegetables and fruit and not any other color of vegetable or fruit. The researchers "found for each 25-g/d increase of white fruit and vegetable consumption a 9% lower risk of stroke".[320] (For each 25-gram intake per day increase they saw a 9% lower risk.)

There are a few white vegetables that are in the cruciferous group of vegetables and have been the focal point for numerous studies. Cruciferous vegetables are very valuable for our health. There is more information on this category of vegetables in the section on green vegetables, since most of the cruciferous vegetables are green.

Here is a list of awesome white vegetables to keep in your diet, white onions, garlic, turnips, ginger, jicama, fennel, cauliflower, kohlrabi, parsnips, potatoes, white asparagus, leeks, daikon, shallots, and mushrooms.

Yellow and orange vegetables get their coloring from carotenoids. Among the different carotenoids, the ones we consume most often are, alpha-carotene, beta-carotene, beta-cryptoxanthin, lycopene, lutein, and zeaxanthin. Alpha-carotene and beta-carotene become

Vitamin A in our bodies. Vitamin A is necessary for proper growth and development, cell differentiation, vision, a healthy immune system, and reproduction. Vitamin A is used by your lungs, kidneys, and heart.

Carotenoids are heart protective due to some effects they have on our bodies. First, carotenoids lower blood pressure, thereby preventing a higher demand on the heart. Second, carotenoids prevent the oxidation of cholesterol in the arteries. Third, carotenoids reduce pro-inflammatory cytokines, which allows for healthier arteries. Fourth, carotenoids are such a powerful antioxidant they make a vital difference in clearing out reactive oxygen species and free radicals, which are both damaging to your arteries, as well as your entire body. Still another great benefit that makes a difference to your heart is that carotenoids facilitate insulin usage, which keeps your blood glucose levels lower, which makes a huge difference to the health of your heart.

Also important is the contribution carotenoids makes to your cells in facilitating cell-to-cell communication. This is an absolute necessity for an organism to stay alive since staying alive requires multiple constant metabolic processes. In other words, there is nothing static about your wonderful human body. There is a constant process of building up of proteins and substances required by your body and simultaneously the breaking down of what no longer serves your body. It's a lot! Cell-to-cell communication has to exist for our organism – us – to be alive. Cell-to-cell communication keeps cells healthy and without it cells can go rogue - as in cancer cells. Cancer cells have lost this ability to communicate to neighboring cells to work in a coordinated fashion for the survival of healthy cells.

Yellow and orange vegetables include butternut squash, spaghetti squash, carrots, yellow winter and summer squash, pumpkin, yellow potatoes, sweet potatoes, and yams. Orange and yellow bell peppers are included in this list even though they are a fruit because they are a great snack, delicious in many meals, and low in fructose. The same goes for yellow tomatoes; they are a fruit but they do not contain as much fructose as other fruits like grapes, bananas, watermelon, etc ... and they are super as a snack.

Red vegetables are most known for their lycopene content (lycopene is a carotenoid). Lycopene is a powerful antioxidant and the focus of many research studies. Most of us have heard of lycopene as the powerhouse phytonutrient in tomatoes. It is known to reduce your risk of some cancers, including breast, renal/kidney, and prostate, which have all been shown to have reduced incidence for people with a high intake of lycopene. The Women's Health Initiative of 1993-1998 and the follow-up in 2013 revealed that for the women that consumed the highest amount of lycopene through their vegetable and fruit intake, those women had fewer cases of renal cancer.[321] Lycopene has been shown to be kidney protective in that it is able to eliminate some medicines that are known to be toxic to the kidneys. Lycopene can reduce your risk of cardiovascular disease, help you fight off infections, and is protective for your eyes.

Red vegetables contain another powerhouse phytonutrient, anthocyanins, which is also a powerful antioxidant. Researchers have discovered more than 635 anthocyanins in nature.[322] The antioxidants in anthocyanins are so powerful they are capable of reducing the chances of developing obesity. Another benefit from the potent anthocyanins is in balancing blood glucose levels, A1c levels, which can help lower your risk of developing metabolic syndrome and type 2 diabetes. For a person that already has type 2 diabetes, anthocyanins are helpful in reducing secondary health problems that usually occur as a result of the diabetes. For all of us it is important to know that anthocyanins are helpful in preventing cardiovascular disease. As if those weren't enough reasons to consume anthocyanins regularly, make a mental note that they are very helpful in lowering the risk of cancers.[323]

Anthocyanins reduce inflammation, reduce blood pressure, are liver protective, and help your vision. Anthocyanins have also been shown to be anti-viral. A few studies have shown that some anthocyanins can cross the blood-brain barrier, thereby playing a role in neuroprotection.[324] [325] The anthocyanins that cross the blood brain barrier have a positive effect to a few of the neurotransmitters and actively influence some biochemical signaling.[326] [327] One more important property of anthocyanins is they promote blood vessel health; this is most likely due to their powerful antioxidant function combined with the anti-inflammatory abilities. The ability of anthocyanins to prevent blood clotting is related to the anti-inflammatory effects. And anthocyanins are helpful to cells by serving to protect them. These are all really good reasons to eat red vegetables several times a week.

Here is a list of some valuable red vegetables, red beets, radicchio, radishes, red leaf lettuce, red onions, red potatoes, and rhubarb qualifies as "red". And again, even though technically red tomatoes and red bell peppers are fruits I will list them here as they are great choices for a snack, and they are scrumptious additions to many different meals.

Purple vegetables provide anthocyanins; this is the phytonutrient responsible for the red and purple color. As already noted, anthocyanins are known as powerful antioxidants, which is likely why they have a strong anti-cancer effect. A study using extracts of anthocyanins found that they inhibited the growth of a human colon cancer cell line.[328] Anthocyanins reduce inflammation, which is very important since inflammation is an environment that is the perfect storm for other diseases to develop. Anthocyanins reduce blood pressure, are liver protective, help your vision, and have some anti-viral abilities.

Studies have also shown that anthocyanins induce apoptosis, which is cell death. Apoptosis is a vital regulatory function of each cell. Each cell is only supposed to live a certain amount of time, and then the programmed cell death is to ensure the cell doesn't become altered and function in an abnormal way, such as cancerous. Cancer is a cell that has been altered, is not functioning normally, but won't die. Anthocyanins promote cell death, which is crucial in preventing cancers from growing.

The high antioxidant activity combined with the ability to induce apoptosis from anthocyanins could be the main reason anthocyanins defend against cancer. Cranberries were studied for their role as a safer anti-cancer therapy.[329] "In recent years, increasing body of evidence has underscored the cancer preventive efficacy of isothiocyanates and anthocyanins in both in vitro and in vivo animal"[330] studies. Another study on tart cherry juice showed an increase in apoptosis in a dose-dependent manner.[331] A study on purple tomatoes, Sun Black tomatoes as they were called, specifically the skin of these tomatoes, was tested against two human cancer cell lines. The result was an inhibition of cancer cell proliferation due to the anthocyanins, in a dose-dependent method.[332] This is just a very small example of some of the studies done on anthocyanins.

Purple vegetables include eggplant, purple kohlrabi, purple bok choy, purple carrots, purple tomatoes, purple potatoes, purple corn, radicchio, purple cabbage, and black olives are considered to be in the purple vegetable family. As these veggies are visually beautiful and make all dishes containing them more appealing – how can you resist?

Chlorophyll is the phytonutrient that makes green vegetables green. It is a strong antioxidant known to be highly effective in eliminating free radicals. Deep green veggies therefore provide anti-cancer benefits, which may also be due in part to chlorophyll's protective effect on DNA, which reduces DNA damage. Liver health is crucial to overall health, and chlorophyll promotes liver health by enhancing the phase II biotransformation enzymes that are responsible for breaking down harmful toxins. Chlorophyll increases the oxygen in our cells so that wounds heal faster. And of course, if there is more oxygen in the cells, brain health is positively affected due to higher oxygen delivery. Another way chlorophyll can help your brain health is because chlorophyll increases red blood cells. The increase in red blood cells is one of the ways green vegetables increases oxygen levels. How can you go wrong if you are eating green right?

Green vegetables also provide lutein, another beneficial

phytonutrient. Lutein benefits your vision, has anti-cancer abilities, and promotes heart health, all of these benefits should sound familiar as they are the benefits derived from carotenoids, and lutein is a carotenoid. Most vegetables that contain lutein also have zeaxanthin, another phytonutrient in green leafy vegetables and also a carotenoid. Studies have shown that lutein and zeaxanthin cross the blood-brain barrier and are very helpful to your brain in reducing cognitive decline. This reduction in cognitive decline is in part through how they help your vision. A study done on middle-aged adults, prior to having any cognitive decline, showed that the greater the amount of lutein and zeaxanthin in their retina, the more neuroprotection their brain had.[333] Wild huh? Actually there are several studies that have determined this relationship so now you know this is not a one-off.

Some of the green vegetables are in the classification of cruciferous vegetables, these are: kale, broccoli, tatsoi, green cabbage, Chinese cabbage, bok choy, rutabaga, arugula, radishes, wasabi, daikon, horseradish, turnips, mustard seeds and leaves, kohlrabi, watercress, Brussels sprouts, and collard greens. There have been numerous studies on cruciferous vegetables and many great results because their benefits are plentiful. Cruciferous vegetables contain a phytonutrient called glucosinolate, which through digestion becomes indoles – thiocyanates, isothiocyanates, and nitriles. Cruciferous vegetables are commonly thought of as anti-cancer, and most of the anti-cancer abilities of deep green vegetables are attributed to these indoles and isothiocyanates. According to the National Cancer Institute, indoles and isothiocyanates are protective against damage to DNA,[334] "help inactivate carcinogens,"[335] have "anti-viral and antibacterial effects,"[336] "have anti-inflammatory effects,"[337] promotes cell death,[338] "inhibits tumor blood vessel formation"[339] and "tumor cell migration"[340] and stops cells from proliferating. [341] Indoles have also been proven to enhance the intestinal epithelial barrier function,[342] acting to keep the contents of the intestines in the intestines as needed.

Quercetin, previously discussed, is another powerful phytonutrient in cruciferous vegetables. Many people think of heart health when they hear the word quercetin as studies have shown a strong benefit to the heart for the following reasons: reduces atherosclerosis, which is the buildup of plaque in the arteries; has strong anti-inflammatory action; and is a very good antioxidant. Put just those three capabilities together and you can see how tremendous quercetin is for your heart. But there is another benefit to the heart and that is the ability of quercetin to lower cholesterol. How amazing is this phyotnutrient?! To keep your heart healthy, eat foods high in quercetin, (which is all vegetables and fruits).

Quercetin helps your body in still more ways. It can help reduce histamine response in allergies and asthma, which are autoimmune conditions. Quercetin can also reduce pain in autoimmune problems like arthritis and fibromyalgia. And, here is the trifecta, quercetin helps with gout. Gout is on the pathogenetic commonality spectrum with rheumatoid arthritis and heart disease, meaning that for the people who have gout, they are at increased risk of getting rheumatoid arthritis and an increased risk of having heart disease. Quercetin is beneficial for all three of these health problems. Isn't that amazing?

Additional and fascinating scientific studies on the cruciferous vegetables have provided other life-changing results. These next two studies concluded the sulforaphane, which is from isothiocyanates in cruciferous vegetables, produces remarkable health benefits. The first of these two studies yielded fascinating results showing the sulforaphane in cruciferous vegetables protected the gastric-intestinal cells from oxidative stress induced from Helicobacter Pylori/H Pylori infection and NSAIDs (non-steroidal anti-inflammatory drugs).[343] The second study will make a difference to people's lives for their future brain health as this study concluded that sulforaphane protected the dopamine neurons in the substantia nigra from deterioration, which can play a role in Parkinson's disease.[344] These two results are head-turners! And think about the ramifications of the health benefits from each study on each other by thinking about the relationship between a healthy intestinal tract and a healthy brain as explained in the chapter "The Gut Microbiota and Your Brain."

As stated, there are a few white vegetables that are cruciferous that confer all the amazing benefits that the green cruciferous vegetables bestow. The white cruciferous vegetables are radishes, turnips, kohlrabi, watercress, rutabagas, and cauliflower.

Green vegetables you should eat are kale, broccoli, collard greens, mustard greens, Brussels sprouts, green cabbage, romaine lettuce, arugula and other lettuces, watercress, celery, bok choy, asparagus, edamame, zucchini, green beans, green onions, spinach, artichokes, leeks, green olives, snap peas, sugar snap peas, and of course, green bell peppers and avocados, even though they are fruits. The green cruciferous vegetables are listed in the previous section about green vegetables.

Green herbs that have important helpful attributes are basil, rosemary, thyme, and oregano. These need to be mentioned as they provide a phytonutrient called triterpinoid that becomes ursolic acid once it has been digested. In studies, ursolic acid has been shown to be anti-inflammatory; anti-fibrotic - it stops the body from producing excess fibrous connective tissue, like scar tissue, or in the case of fibromyalgia; anti-proliferative, it stops cells from reproducing at a rapid rate, like cancer cells; anti-angiogenesis, it stops cells from creating their own blood vessel formation, like cancer cells do in order to survive.[345] These herbs can easily be added into many bean dishes, pasta, potato dishes, salads, soups, dressings, and rice dishes.

Cilantro and parsley are also herbs and, like the green vegetables, contain chlorophyll. It is easy to add both cilantro and parsley into many foods to increase your dose of chlorophyll. You can put them into salad dressings, salads, guacamole, green juices, pastas, rice dishes, soups, and make pesto with them.

For all the above reasons, you should make it a priority to eat green vegetables at least five days a week. If you consistently eat green vegetables at this rate for one year, you will feel much better for it. Green vegetables pack a high amount of nutrients and are hard to beat as one of the top foods you should be eating.

The Sum Is Greater Than the Individual Parts: Superfoods

When it comes to vegetables, the sum of the parts is greater than the individual components. The sum, the combination of all the phytonutrients, is much bigger than the individual phytonutrients. The pharmaceutical industry would love to be able to create a pill that could do all the things that even one vegetable does for you. But, it is not possible because man-made substances do not have the same effects that plants have. And vegetables have positive side effects.

Another thing the pharmaceutical industry can't do is create 1 pill that would positively affect a few organs, the blood, and the brain. But every vegetable does that. Every vegetable contributes to create a healthy intestinal tract, healthy liver, strong immune system, healthy hormonal system, healthy blood vessels, and healthier brain. So you don't need a pill to promote your health-you need vegetables. What follows is a list of the superfoods and the extraordinary benefits from them. This is not a complete list of the benefits from vegetables to our bodies, and does not include the individual benefits of each vegetable.

It is a package deal. And a great one at that! Numerous studies have determined that every vegetable that has obtained "Superfood" status did so specifically because of its cumulative benefits. Every superfood can be broken down into its phytonutrient content and its many benefits. It is a great package deal! Each superfood has been the focus of numerous research studies, which is why we have all of this important and life-enhancing information. There is no better way to give your body exactly what it needs than feeding it superfoods.

Superfood broccoli is one of the cruciferous vegetables. Packaged in broccoli is a large dose of fiber; powerful antioxidants; and the phytonutrients zeaxanthin and lutein, which have tremendous benefits to your vision. Deep green vegetables have shown to be helpful in reducing colon cancer due to the phytonutrient's indoles and isothiocyanates. Another contributing factor in lowering colon cancer risk is the high fiber content. While another huge factor is the phytonutrients supplying the liver what it needs to be able to produce the phase 2 detoxification enzymes that reduce toxic bio-chemical production. Broccoli also has quercetin, which increases the beneficial effects of the other phytonutrients.

Kale, another cruciferous vegetable, achieved superfood status because of its numerous benefits. It's regarded highly as an anti-cancer vegetable due to a few of the actions it has in the body. Its anti-cancer benefits extend to protection against intestinal, breast and ovarian cancers. Its high-fiber content increases its value for the intestines and also serves to keep blood sugar levels low. Keeping blood sugar levels low is also important with regards to reducing risk for cancer since high blood sugar levels induce other bioactive pathways and growth factors that are seen in people with cancers. Kale's quercetin content super-charges its other phytonutrients, making it the superfood it is. It is hard to overstate how good kale is for you.

Spinach is another cruciferous vegetable that is also a superfood. The vitamins and phytonutrients contained in spinach make it a powerful antioxidant. Looking at the synergistic effects from the phytonutrients in spinach it is hard to top spinach as a superfood. Synergistically, the minerals in spinach help stabilize blood pressure and keep the heart rate low, combine that with the effect from a whopping does of fiber to keep cholesterol low and it's easy to see why regular consumption of spinach would be great for your heart. As a cruciferous vegetable, spinach also has quercetin which, again, bolsters the efficacy of the other phytonutrients making it a food that you should eat often. Now look at the combined benefits from the fiber, it is very good for your intestines by providing substrate for healthy organisms to develop from, and reduces colon cancer risk. Also, all that fiber is great for your entire body as it helps prevent metabolic syndrome and diabetes by stabilizing blood sugar levels. Preventing metabolic syndrome and diabetes protects your heart as both of these health problems negatively impact heart health. Spinach is rich in the phytonutrients lutein, zeaxanthin, and B-carotene, which all contribute to maintaining good vision. Zeaxanthin also helps to reduce the risk of age-related macular degeneration.

Avocados are a superfood because they are anti-inflammatory, supply healthy fats, lots of fiber, and carotenoids. This combination of reduced inflammation, healthy fats, fiber, and carotenoids contribute to your heart health in a number of ways: Low levels of inflammation usually contributes to keeping blood pressure low which is helpful to your heart. The healthy fats lower the risk of heart disease and combined with the effect of keeping blood pressure low is a win-win for your heart. The fiber helps your heart in several ways: it keep cholesterol low, helps to keep the healthy HDL cholesterol up, and keeps blood glucose/A1c levels low, which reduces your chances of getting metabolic syndrome and type 2 diabetes, which negatively affect your heart. The carotenoids provide powerful antioxidants, which prevent oxidation of cholesterol, making them important for your heart health by lowering your risk of developing cardiovascular disease. Synergistically the effects from avocados to your heart are tremendous.

Your brain also benefits from the combination of reduced inflammation, healthy fats, fiber, and carotenoids. Reduced inflammation supports the integrity of your blood brain barrier while inflammation alters it. Additionally, the reduced inflammation leads to lower blood pressure and just as low blood pressure is helpful to your heart, it is also beneficial for your brain. The healthy fats are needed for your brain and help reduce your risk of stroke. While you can think of these two effects as also helping each other to maintain brain health – lower blood pressure reduces stroke risk and so does healthy fats. The fiber helps your brain health by reducing brain inflammation which lowers your risk of cognitive decline with age, memory loss as well as neurodegenerative processes. Carotenoids have antioxidants, which help in lowering your chance of getting certain cancers. Avocados' anti-inflammatory benefits also contribute to reducing cancers. The combination of all these benefits for your brain health is important.

Onions should be included in your diet often as they have many protective benefits. Organosulfur compounds in onions are known to reduce the histamine response, so therefore are helpful for people with allergies. The organosulfur compounds can help combat certain bacteria. Onions also have anti-clotting abilities to ensure that blood is not clotting unnecessarily, that is, enough to close a wound but not so much to impede blood flow. The phytonutrients quercetin and kaempferol in onions have noteworthy anti-cancer properties. Several studies on onions have shown an inverse relationship of onion consumption and a reduced risk for cancers at several different body sites. Cumulatively, the ability to stop blood from forming unnecessary clots and having the ability to ward off cancer works hand-in-hand as cancer can be thought of as an extreme case of blood stasis. Chronic systemic inflammation is blood stasis, exemplifying that if onions reduce clotting they reduce inflammation.

Studies have shown numerous very helpful effects from garlic intake putting it on the superfood list. Garlic increases the body's immune response. It causes an increase in Natural Killer (NK) cells,[346] whose function is to survey for bacteria, viruses, and tumorous cells and cause them to die. Garlic has been shown to increase the number of NK cells in the lymph nodes.[347] Garlic reduces the inflammatory response, which is very important in metabolic syndrome, diabetes, obesity, cardiovascular disease, and some digestive disorders, and it is able to ward off some cancer strains.[348] Garlic is a very effective antioxidant.[349] As an example of the sum being greater than the individual parts: the antioxidant properties in garlic are very helpful in metabolic syndrome, diabetes, obesity, cardiovascular disease, some digestive disorders, and cancers, every one of these diseases manifests chronic systemic inflammation which garlic is also very helpful in reducing. This cumulative effect is very powerful.

I put celery in the superfood group for one specific reason - it helps change damage caused by lipopolysaccharides, or LPS. The flavones in celery, called apigenin, can change a situation that especially affects the elderly. LPS are part of the outer membrane of gram-negative bacteria, and in humans they produce fever, cause inflammation and pain, and have a negative effect to liver health. LPS are even a contributing factor in sepsis. LPS is not a bacterium, and antibiotics do not remove LPS from your body. As a result, an infection can leave LPS in your body, affecting your liver, brain, blood vessels, immune system (often causing autoimmune problems), hormones, and intestinal tract. Removing LPS from the body, especially in the elderly, can make a big difference to their health. Though all people who contract a bacterial infection from a gram-negative bacterium will acquire LPS as the bacteria sheds it, the elderly appear to be even more susceptible as they suffer from more frequent infections. Whether someone is tending toward older or is a young person, anyone who gets multiple infections a year has a microbiome that has unhealthy organisms, which allow these infections to occur. And, the more infections, the higher the chances of having infections from gram-negative bacteria which means the higher the levels of accumulated LPS as they do continue to accumulate as they persist in the body even after the infection is gone.

The Sum Is Greater Than the Individual Parts for All Vegetables

Superfoods reached super-star status because each provides multiple healthful benefits to the body accomplished via a synergy of actions and multiple phytonutrients in each. Now think of the cumulative effect of *all* the phytonutrients from *all* the different vegetables too as having a bigger effect than just one individual vegetable. This is what you get from the combination of different vegetables you eat in one meal and you can also think of the different vegetables you eat over the course of one day all having a cumulative effect. That is what is seen in studies. Numerous studies have shown that the higher the vegetable and fruit consumption, the lower the risk of overall mortality. The result from the EPIC 13-year study in Europe was a decreased risk of death for the people who ate 569 grams each day of vegetables and fruit. People who consumed this much had a decreased risk of death due to circulatory, respiratory, and digestive problems.[350] It was also observed that the higher intake of vegetables, not fruit, produced the inverse relationship to those health problems.

The PURE study was an epidemiological study in 18 countries over a 10-year period. The study had 135,335 participants from the full range of low to high income, aged 35-70, and without cardiovascular disease at the beginning of the study. The conclusion reached from observing eating patterns over 10 years was, "Higher total fruit, vegetable, and legume intake was inversely associated with major cardiovascular disease, myocardial infarction, cardiovascular mortality, non-cardiovascular mortality, and total mortality in the models adjusted for age, sex, and centre".[351] The take-away from this study: eating higher amounts of fruit, vegetables, and legumes every day lowered the risk from all-cause-mortality as well as non-cardiovascular death; and eating three to four servings of fruit, vegetables, and legumes every day was enough to make the difference in those health outcomes.[352] This is useful information that you should apply to your life in order to prevent development of the leading causes of death. A study that looked at the top causes of death in 188 countries from the years 1990-2013 determined that the "Cardiometabolic diseases including coronary heart disease (CHD), stroke, and type 2 diabetes are leading causes of morbidity and mortality globally."[353]

In 2011, there was "an unprecedented high-level summit convened by the United Nations (UN) to discuss a critical new global agenda."[354] The need for this unprecedented meeting was the incredible rise in incidence and global threat to health from non-communicable diseases. This is a statement from this meeting: "The primary goal of the summit was to mobilize commitment to confront the worldwide threat posed by four 'globally relevant' noncommunicable diseases (NCDs) — cardiovascular disease, cancer, diabetes, and chronic respiratory disease — and their associated risk factors: tobacco use, unhealthy diet, insufficient physical activity, and harmful use of alcohol."[355] "In 2011, the United Nations highlighted suboptimal diet as one of the principal drivers of these diseases".[356] Two of the greatest risk factors to our health are lifestyle factors, factors we have control over, our diet and our physical activity; though we actually have control over our tobacco use and alcohol intake too.

An important point to keep in mind is the value of antioxidants in vegetables and fruits. All vegetables and fruits have antioxidants, which are needed to neutralize reactive oxygen species, or ROS, to prevent the damage done to cells by the ROS. All diseases have high rates of ROS. (This was discussed in the chapter "Your Microbiome Affects Your Liver and Your Liver Affects Your Microbiome.")

Technology has unlocked the presence and functions of phytonutrients. We now know that it's not just the vitamins and minerals in vegetables and fruits that our bodies require; our bodies require phytonutrients. Thinking wholistically, you can now see how there is a synergistic effect from the array of vitamins, minerals, fiber, and phyotnutrients. This is why it is to your benefit to consume a rainbow of the vegetables available.

Speaking of phytonutrients and vitamins brings up an important point, you are much better off getting the vitamins and phytonutrients your body needs from foods, not from supplements. When you get vitamins from foods, your body can easily utilize them because they have naturally formed molecular structures that are easily broken down and used by your cells. Also, they are in a proportion that is appropriate for the needs of your body.

195

As just discussed, each vegetable offers several phytonutrients and it is the pairs of phytonutrients that often work together synergistically. This fact is why vegetables successfully provide our bodies with the phytonutrients that perfectly fill the demands our cells need. Very importantly also is the fiber that you will get by eating vegetables versus taking a supplement of the phytonutrients and/or vitamins that does not supply your body with the fiber and its numerous benefits.

In 1820, the pharmaceutical industry started making pharmaceutical drugs from the phytonutrients in plants. (This will be discussed in more detail in the chapter "Plants Used as Pharmaceuticals".) That set the stage for the supplement industry to later make dietary supplements of the phytonutrients.
Some supplements on the market have been based on the individual phytonutrients, such as lutein, lycopene, zeaxanthin, and carotenoids. While users may receive some benefits from them, there are a few problems with this model of extracting just one element from a plant.

First, in a number of studies that have isolated what was thought to be the active ingredient from a vegetable, that singled-out active ingredient was given to people, but does not always give the desired results. This is likely because when that phytonutrient is consumed via the plant that is produced from nature, there are other phytonutrients in that vegetable that work in conjunction with the one isolated phytonutrient thought to be the star. The research showed that it is a package-deal: multiple phytonutrients working together provide the health benefits.

Second, another reason for most likely getting less than

desired results from a singled-out phyotnutrient is the bio-availability. Bioavailability is a consequence of which microbes are living in an individual's intestines that are capable of absorbing the phyotnutrients from the foods eaten (this was discussed earlier). A person with a long history of eating processed foods usually has unhealthy bacterial strains, which will not absorb all the phytonutrients that are available from vegetables. But this can be improved upon by simply eating vegetables and fruits to create a healthy gut microbiota. Progressively, as more vegetables are eaten, the intestines develop health-promoting strains of bacteria. As more of the healthy strains of bacteria develop, then more of the phytonutrients from the vegetables can get extracted. You cannot get all the amazing benefits that plants can give you from any one pill! But what you will get from plants is Only phytonutrients that your body needs. And will put to good use to make you the best you can be!

Note that herbs, even in dried form, are still the whole plant. They are not one isolated phytonutrient from a plant, which is why dried herbs do make great changes in the body.

Another bonus from eating several servings of vegetables every day is weight loss. Studies have shown that the people with the highest consumption of vegetables don't put on as much weight as people with lower vegetable consumption. Part of this is attributed to the amounts of fiber people intake with that higher vegetable consumption.

Across the board, thousands of studies have shown the effects from phytonutrients and better health is the result of higher consumption of a *variety* of vegetables - that is what confers the greatest health benefits. It's not eating just one serving a day of vegetables at dinner. It is about eating three to four servings of vegetables every day, as well as eating a variety of fruits. You can even eat veggies for or with your breakfast. It actually is a great way to start your brain off for the day. Give it try, you will most likely find you are able to focus your brain easier - definitely easier than if you have any type of sugar in the morning.

Why is variety so important? As already discussed, eating a variety of vegetables is important so that your intestinal microbiota will develop a diversified range of healthy bacteria. Variety also provides your body with a range of different phytonutrients. Now that you know the strong points from the phytonutrients you can understand how you hedge your bets toward your health when you consistently supply your body with all the phytonutrients, giving you protection on all fronts.

What's the Deal With Short-Chain Fatty Acids?

Your gut-endocrine system is responsible for more functions than any other organ or gland. It directs neurotransmitters; hormones; inflammation; autoimmune reactions, such as allergies and autoimmune diseases; and has an effect to all your other organs. The body, in all its wisdom, is set up like this for reasons. Your gut-endocrine system is entrusted with your energy supply, your energy storage, and your immune system balance. Think about it, your gut is in charge of whether energy is used from the calories you consume or if those calories get put into storage, or whether insulin will effectively carry glucose into your cells. And one more critical piece of information regarding your gut-endocrine system that you need to know about to take control of your health is the short-chain fatty acids and why you should deliberately consume them every day.

You will be hearing more about short-chain fatty acids, or SCFAs, over the next few years, as research on them is still in its infancy. However as researchers are discovering more about them we do already know it is crucial for us to be getting them in our diets. We are learning that our health depends on them. SCFAs play a vital role in either maintaining our health or, in their absence, contributing to the development of disease.

There are three main SCFAs: butyrate, propionate, and acetate. At this point research has been able to tease out some of the specific jobs each has in your body, and in the next decade will provide more details. SCFAs are readily available to everyone as you can easily eat them everyday just by eating vegetables, fruits, nuts, and grains. Our bodies get SCFAs from fermentable fiber - the partially and non-digestible fiber in plants. It's that simple. But what SFCAs do for our bodies is not that simple, but in fact - incredible!

SCFAs control two very important signaling systems that each in turn are catalysts for subsequent actions in the body, which then have numerous downstream effects. One of the signaling systems SCFAs control is the inhibition of histone deacetylases, which is very important for gene regulation; brain plasticity; intestinal cell integrity; as well as gut microbiota-host tolerance, or the ability of the host's immune system to allow commensal bacteria to live in the intestines. The inhibition of histone deacetylases in the intestinal tract is important for anti-inflammatory and anti-proliferation effects to the intestines.

The other major signaling system SCFAs control is the G-protein-coupled receptors, a signaling system that has numerous responses in the body. Here is a brief overview of some of the jobs of the G-protein-coupled receptors: they are a vital component in immune cells; are important for proper immune system response via their anti-inflammatory action; regulate proper immune activity and inhibit autoimmune activity; help reduce colon cancer via their anti-proliferation effects; play a role in gut hormones, allowing you to feel satiated or hungry; affect your metabolism; and affect your ability to use insulin or being insulin resistant.

The control of signaling systems is just a piece of what the SCFAs do. Together the SCFAs are important in maintaining the mucosal barrier of the intestines, thereby preventing food and the breakdown from foods to get leaked out of the intestinal tube. SCFAs are needed also for their regulation over the immune system. And another irreplaceable function of the SCFAs is their signaling to a specific protein, inducing the repair and maintenance of the inner layer of cells throughout your entire GI tract.[357] [358] As a whole, the SCFAs are absolutely necessary if you want to have a healthy digestive tract, which now we know is not just digestive health but overall health.

While there is much more to discover about the SCFAs and there will be wonderful new information about them in the coming years, it is a fact right now that if you increase your SCFA intake through vegetables today and continue daily to eat vegetables three to five times a day, since you can eat them with every meal and also as snacks, you will improve your health. Our bodies need all of the SCFAs for each of the functions they carry out in our bodies. Let's take a look at each individual SCFA for its specific effects.

Let's take a look at butyrate first. Most of the butyrate you get from the vegetables you eat is actually consumed by the cells in your intestines to supply them with energy.[359]

An analogy would be either gasoline or electricity for your car. Without the needed energy source, your car will not move or otherwise function just as the right fuel/energy source must be available for the cells in the intestines to function. Without a consistent source of butyrate/fuel, the cells in the intestinal tract will not function, leading to disease. You can also think of this as a barter system. Healthy cells in your intestines function to maintain your health; in exchange they take a percentage of butyrate to feed themselves. Sounds fair to me!

When the cells in the intestinal tract are not healthy, they cannot fight off invading pathogenic bacteria. This has been seen in a number of studies where the researchers saw that the presence of butyrate helps fight off pathogenic bacteria. Butyrate in your intestinal tract stimulates production of proteins that fight off pathogenic types of organisms.[360] This explains how butyrate protects against the development of colitis. This is evidenced now by the vast number of studies showing that people with irritable bowel syndrome,[361] inflammatory bowel disease,[362], colitis,[363] and even Crohn's disease[364] all have low levels of butyrate. A study done in 2006 saw that butyrate promoted the growth of the healthy bacterial strains of lactobacilli and bifidobacteria in the large intestines[365] and these healthy strains defend their territory. This is the contrast to the many studies that have seen very low levels of SCFAs in people with inflammatory bowel disease,[366] [367] irritable bowel syndrome,[368] Crohn's disease, and colitis.[369] An improvement of these digestive disorders has been seen upon administration of the SCFAs.[370] [371]

Numerous studies have observed an altered microbiota in patients who are critically ill and in the intensive care unit. The consensus is that the gut microbiota in this group is low in butyrate. And several studies have shown that this population also has reduced levels of all the SCFAs compared to the general population. Butyrate is significantly lower in the critically ill population. This is crucial since butyrate is *the* number one fuel source for the cells in the colon and if butyrate levels are low to non-existent, the health of the intestinal cells will be affected negatively. Also crucial is that butyrate has a cell-protective effect for colon cells. It keeps the colon cells healthy and functioning optimally, which is connected to its effect of reducing intestinal inflammation. As it's all about the real estate (as explained earlier), butyrate competes with pathogenic bacteria by not allowing them to thrive, or by making it hard for them to implant and thrive.

As you have just read, butyrate plays a role in protecting the cells in the colon, and one of the functions involved with this protection is through its induction of cell death to cells that are old, damaged, or not functioning.[372] Causing cell death is preventive in reducing colo-rectal cancer risk by removing cells that can potentially become cancerous. You will recall from earlier in this chapter that SCFAs control one of the signaling systems called histone deacetylases, and this is another way butyrate acts preventively against colo-rectal cancer. Signaling through the histone deacetylase system inhibits cellular proliferation, thereby reducing the chances of getting colo-rectal cancer - another way butyrate reduces potential danger to the intestinal tract.[373]

Here is another absolutely fascinating gut-brain connection: butyrate is carried to and seen in abundance at the blood-brain barrier. It is thought that butyrate crosses the blood-brain barrier and serves as "a major energy source in cellular metabolism"[374] for brain cells. Taking this a step further - since we have already seen the connection between a healthy intestinal barrier and its impact to your blood-brain barrier, and since we know that butyrate is a needed factor in maintaining the intestinal barrier - some researchers have seen that the SCFAs butyrate and propionate also play a significant role in maintaining your blood-brain barrier.[375]

Butyrate also increases metabolism, helping to expend calories, thereby playing a role in weight. Directly related to that is butyrate's role in reducing the risk of getting metabolic syndrome,[376] which has been seen in several studies. Consuming several SCFAs daily can lower your risk of getting metabolic syndrome. Think back for a moment, recall that anthocyanins, and anthocyanidins help combat obesity and are very good at helping prevent metabolic syndrome and type 2 diabetes, as is butyrate. The thought is that if you consume vegetables high in anthocyanins, and anthocyanidins you will get the butyrate your body needs and the compounded benefits of each of these three which help in reducing chances of obesity and reducing risk of metabolic syndrome and type 2 diabetes.

Propionate is taken up in your liver where it helps the liver to make glucose, or fuel, from the foods you eat. Propionate in your liver also helps to store fuel. And, it is very important in influencing your cholesterol levels, as it reduces the rate at which your liver makes cholesterol.[377]

Research has also shown that propionate plays an important role in the integrity of the blood-brain barrier. One group of researchers saw that propionate "inhibited pathways associated with non-specific microbial infections"; protected the brain from the lipopolysaccharides from bacteria that often affects the brain when someone has an infection; and propionate protected the brain from oxidative stress.[378]

Acetate is the most abundant SCFA and is involved in several critical processes that affect your health. It is delivered to peripheral tissues where it plays a role in cholesterol synthesis. Acetate is found in the cerebrospinal fluid.[379] And it is found in the brain where it provides fuel for brain cells.[380] One of the known effects from acetate to your brain is on appetite suppression.[381] Acetate is also required if you want to have a healthy intestinal tract as shown through its promotion of IgA,[382] an antibody that specializes in protecting intestinal cells.[383]

There is another practical connection you can make here with regards to the SCFA and the incomparable effects for your brain health. Since butyrate and propionate are vital for your blood brain barrier and acetate is the food for your brain cells, you would help your brain health by increasing your vegetable intake.

These are all good reasons that should be catalysts to inspire you to eat SCFAs every day.

SCFAs have also been implicated in heart health as researchers have noted the direct effect from the gut microbiota to heart health as well as the direct relationship of the SCFAs to heart health. It has been known for decades that high blood pressure is one of the strongest risk factors for developing cardiovascular disease, and by maintaining a healthy blood pressure level you reduce your risk of progressing to it. In 2017, a controlled trial in people resulted in achieving a reduction in diastolic blood pressure from the use of butyrate.[384] (Diastolic blood pressure is the reading of the pressure in your arteries when your heart relaxes between contractions. It is represented by the number under the slash, or in the lower position.) And while butyrate is helpful in reducing inflammation which then has the effect of lowering blood pressure, all the SCFAs play a role in your heart health.[385] There are currently many researchers who have stated that the future of cardiovascular medicine must look at the influence the gut microbiota and SCFAs have to the heart.[386] [387] [388] [389] These are but a few examples out of many that determined this relationship between the SCFAs and the impact to the heart.

Currently there are a good number of studies proving the impact of SCFAs, but, we only get SCFAs by consuming foods that have fiber. SCFAs and dietary fiber are a package-deal. The foods that supply this fiber are non-digestible plants - vegetables, fruit, grains, and legumes. When you eat plants, the fiber supplies the substrates that the microorganisms ferment, which then produce the SCFAs. We have already looked at the SCFAs, now let's look at how fiber affects us and why we need it.

Hundreds of scientific studies all consistently point out that dietary fiber and the SCFAs are necessary in our diets in order to prevent a number of diseases. Data from the 2009-2010 National Health and Nutrition Examination Study revealed that Americans were consuming about 16.2 grams of fiber on a daily basis.[390] This is only half of the recommended range of 28-30 grams per day for adults by the American Heart Association/American College of Cardiology.[391] The goal for which this range for fiber intake was created states: "By 2020, to improve the cardiovascular health of all Americans by 20% while reducing deaths from cardiovascular diseases and stroke by 20%."[392] Through hundreds of studies and years worth of epidemiological studies we know that dietary fiber lowers the risk of cardio-vascular disease.[393] [394] [395] [396] [397]

Earlier chapters in this book provide a good amount of information on obesity and its relationship to your microbiota, to food additives and artificial sweeteners, to autoimmune activation, to hormonal changes, to your liver health, and to how vegetables can make a difference. What hasn't been discussed yet is the role fiber plays in obesity. There are hundreds of studies proving the relationship of fiber intake and the SCFAs to obesity.[398] [399] [400] [401] These studies show there is an inverse relationship of fiber consumption and obesity - the higher the fiber intake, the lower the chances of being obese.

There are several biochemical reactions that occur when you eat fiber. Each of these, as well as the synergistic effect of all of them in your body, explains why this inverse relationship of fiber and weight exists.

One reason is that fiber is bulky and absorbs water, which causes stomach distension. This distension sends a signal through your vagus nerve to your brain informing your brain your stomach is getting filled up. Fiber-rich foods are more viscous, and this viscosity slows down the rate of gastric emptying. While the stomach is full for a longer length of time the vagus nerve continues to signal to your brain that it still has food and eating is not required. Another reaction that occurs when you eat fiber is that most fiber requires more chewing. The more you have to chew, the slower you will eat, which usually means you will be eating for a longer period of time. A prolonged time of slow eating exposes your brain to a longer duration of satiety signals telling your brain that you are no longer hungry. Another biochemical reaction that happens when you eat fiber is the production of acetate, which gets transported to the hypothalamus, which then signals to your brain that you are no longer hungry.

Another health problem you know about that is plaguing America currently is type 2 diabetes, and here too, fiber intake is a crucial dietary factor that makes the difference with regards to developing or not developing type 2 diabetes. Numerous studies on fiber have seen an inverse association between high dietary fiber intake through vegetables and fruit and a reduced incidence of type 2 diabetes.[402][403][404][405] It's hard to argue with such consistent results.

Let's look at the relationships among the three health problems just discussed: cardiovascular disease, obesity, and type 2 diabetes mellitus, or T2DM. In doing so, realize that the majority of cases for each of these health problems is a lifestyle disease, which means- preventable for most of the people that have one or all of them. Also realize that here too we are looking at pathogenetic commonalities (discussed earlier in the chapter "Everything Old Is New Again") refers to the spectrum of one disease connecting it to the propensity to develop one or more diseases due to shared pathological processes and disease progression. Obesity is a risk factor for developing T2DM. Epidemiological and scientific studies all draw the correlation of a greater incidence rate of T2DM in people who are obese. Having obesity and T2DM increases the chances of developing cardiovascular problems. These three health problems are connected because of their shared negative effects to the body. They are each the progression of an altered microbiome on a one-way course. By contrast, the positive benefits from the SCFAs are also connected by interacting through several biochemical processes that maintain a healthy body.

To be healthy, your body needs the three main SCFAs, butyrate, propionate and acetate. Without them there are health problems that will progress and develop into more and worsening health problems. The fiber that is absolutely necessary if you want to be healthy is part of the package deal when you consume the SCFAs - think of it as a double-bonus!

It's really simple – eat more vegetables to be healthy!

Plants Used as Pharmaceuticals

Plants have been used as the basis for pharmaceutical medications since 1820 when quinine from the bark of the cinchona tree was isolated and used for malaria. It had been used to treat malaria in Europeans since 1638, as it was brought in from South America, however it was only used in its natural form, meaning the bark was dried, ground, and mixed into liquid for use. (This is still one method of using herbs today.) Though before the quinine was isolated in 1820, native people in other countries had been using it in its natural form for centuries for ailments.

In 1826, morphine was derived from the poppy plant. Aspirin was developed from the bark of the White Willow tree in 1899. In 1250, writings from a Flemish family describe their use of digitalis for heart conditions.[406] Digitalis from the foxglove plant continued to be used for heart and other problems until 1930, at which time Digoxin first became isolated and put to use, as it still is, as a pharmaceutical drug for cardiovascular problems.

The term "pharmacognosy" came into use in the 19th

century, referring to the drugs that were based on natural substances, such as plants, animals, and minerals. Now "pharmacognosy" as defined by the American Society of Pharmacognosy is "the study of the physical, chemical, biochemical and biological properties of drugs, drug substances or potential drugs or drug substances of natural origin as well as the search for new drugs from natural sources".[407]

The study of plants for human health is currently thriving. While it's well known that herbs and plants have been in use for thousands of years for health purposes, many do not know of the history of plants used in pharmaceutical medications or that plants are still used today as the basis for a large number of the drugs that are currently manufactured. "For example, from 1981 to 2010, natural products and their derivatives were the source of 41% of new drugs and 79.8% of all approved anticancer drugs."[408]

From 2000-2010, 50% of the new drugs being tested actually came in to existence because the active component of those drugs was either a natural compound or derived from a natural compound. Some of these compounds were taken from plants, algae, bacteria, or fungi. The vital role that nature plays in the current pharmaceutical industry cannot be overstated. Plants, algae, bacteria, and fungi provide molecular structures that have very helpful effects to our bodies. Natural products and the derivatives that scientists make from them are the basis for the majority of anti-infective medications and drugs used to combat cancer. Natural products are the basis for drugs for other diseases as well: cardiovascular issues; immunosuppressant drugs for autoimmune problems; anti-parasitic drugs; and anti-diabetic drugs.

Many researchers and scientists today know how vital natural products are for their role in new drug development. In 2015, the Nobel Prize for the category "Physiology or Medicine" was won by three scientists who discovered and helped develop natural sources into medicines that are making a difference in two huge health crisis' that affects millions of people in developing countries. Professor Tu won half of the Nobel Prize for her discovery and development of the drug Artemisinin, from the sweet wormwood plant, which combats malaria. The other half of the 2015 Nobel Prize went to Drs. Omura and Campbell for their discovery and development of the drug Ivermectin, which fights several parasites effecting millions of people in Africa.

"Even at the dawn of 21st century, 11% of the 252 drugs considered as basic and essential by the WHO (World Health Organization) were exclusively of flowering plant origin."[409] This is amazing to realize because as far as we have come in advancing medicine, this shows that nature is crucial to Western Medicine and crucial for our health.

If you still think plants can't actually change conditions in your body, and if you are a coffee or tea drinker, ask yourself why you drink that beverage. Does it stimulate you? These two highly popular drinks are from plants, coffee from a bean and tea from leaves. If they didn't really cause stimulation, do you think they would be as popular as they are?

A 2001 article by two researchers stated: "We have identified 122 compounds of defined structure, obtained from only 94 species of plants, that are used globally as drugs and demonstrate that 80% of these have had an ethnomedical use identical or related to the current use of the active elements of the plant."[410] (Ethnomedical is traditional medicine that encompasses the range of health care practiced by indigenous people from different cultures dating back thousands of years.) This is very telling as it conveys that "80%"[411] of the drugs made from or based on plants to treat some medical problems today are the same plants used to treat the same problems among indigenous people thousands of years ago and in some situations still today. At the time of this writing, there are over 200 patents in process to the FDA to make medications from plants.

Since natural products are still a very important contributor to the pharmaceutical industry, there are two doctors who started an informative review of natural products in pharmacology, feeling it was important to have this reference. Dr. David J. Newman, retired from the National Institute of Cancer, and Dr. Gordon M. Cragg have compiled a log that is keeping track of all the pharmaceutical drugs that are from natural products, based on natural products and their derivatives. Their research reveals that from 1981-2010, out of the 1,355 newly produced medications in all countries only "29% were synthetic in origin, thus demonstrating the influence of 'other than formal synthetics' on drug discovery and approval."[412] In 2014, 10 out of 44 new drugs produced were either natural, or based on natural substance, representing 25% of the new drugs produced in 2014.[413] Between 2000-2008, about 40% of the new drugs produced were either natural products or based on natural products.[414] When it comes to drugs for cancer, from about the 1940s until 2014 "of the 175 small molecules, 131, or 74.8%, are other than "S" (synthetic), with 85, or 48.6%, actually being either natural products or directly derived there from."[415]

In the first review from Drs. Newman and Cragg, *Natural Products as Sources of New Drugs Over the 30 Years From 1981 to 2010,* in their conclusion, the two Drs. state that their colleagues have voiced their opinions to the researchers telling them that they believe that giving credit to the natural product from which the active compound is used for a drug to be developed from "is an overstatement of the role played by natural products in the drug discovery process."[416] The authors of the review state this: "On the contrary, we would still argue that these further serve to illustrate the inspiration provided by Nature to receptive organic chemists in devising ingenious syntheses of structural mimics to compete with Mother Nature's longstanding substrates."[417]

I appreciate that Drs. Newman and Cragg were candid and wrote these responses from their colleagues. First, it is important to give credit where credit is due, which the researchers themselves do. If a drug becomes a drug as the result of an active component from a natural substance, that natural product deserves to be credited. It was due to the existence of that natural compound in the first place that any chemist was able to experiment with its molecular structure to make a drug from it at all.

Secondly, it shows the mindset of "us against them," that is Western medicine vs. natural medicine (acupuncturists, herbalists, chiropractors, naturopaths) still exists in the field of medicine. This does not encompass every professional in the field of Western medicine; there are many doctors, nurses, pharmacists, and researchers who have open minds and can see that natural modalities do make huge contributions to peoples' health. Why is there even a competition? Shouldn't the health profession be about just helping people get better? And since the pharmaceutical industry can see so clearly that natural substances are extremely beneficial, why is there a competition?

Drs. Newman and Cragg are completely on board with crediting natural sources. Through their years of experience and research they have seen how effective natural substances are and still today how many drugs are from or based on natural products. Their statement for organic chemists to see nature as potential to create new drugs is their acknowledgement of the powerful effects natural substances have for humans. I perceive their statement as Mother Nature has set a very high bar with her "longstanding substrates,"[418] which is thousands of years of use by humans.

Nature itself, that is, anything that is alive today be it plant, organism, animal, or human, is still alive because it has evolved and adapted to its environment and fought to stay alive. It is specifically those factors that keep any plant alive that are the crucial components that are beneficial for us. The compounds plants produce to protect themselves from extinction are these phytonutrients that are vital to our health.

We have just entered a new era for research into plants. The same throughput technology that is allowing scientists and researchers to look into the microbiotas in our bodies and see the relationships among different organisms is doing the same for scientists and researchers looking into plants. Since even the 18th century it's been known that there are organisms that live on and in plants. Starting in the early part of the 19th century, it was discovered that different types of fungi lived on plants. Later in the 19th century it was discovered that other types of organisms lived on plants, bacteria, protists, archaea (this should sound familiar - these are the types of organisms that live in and on our bodies discussed at the very beginning of this book). Currently it is well known that plants house numerous types of organisms and when those organisms are mutualistic, they benefit the plant and confer abilities to it, helping it thrive and survive. (This should also sound familiar- as this describes the same type of mutualistic relationship with organisms that we need in our intestinal tract to support a healthy gut). What is new and owing to technology is the ability to see how these organisms affect the plant; it is a new and exciting arena and is filled with potential for helping humans.

If you felt like you were reading a Sci-Fi book in the chapter "Your Microbiome Affects Your Liver & Your Liver Affects Your Microbiome" then hold on tight because here is some more mind-blowing information about plants that also seems to be straight from a Sci-Fi book. All the different polyphenols in plants have developed as a result of the plants' environment and its microbiome - yes, even plants have microbiomes. Just like us, the organisms in and on the plants have a direct impact to the life and health of that plant. These organisms produce metabolites that affect the plant, some of which are protective some of which are threats to the plant's existence.

Many of the polyphenols that are beneficial for our heath are also beneficial to the plant. These polyphenols developed to protect that plant. They are adaptive responses from each plant that allow it to survive. Some examples of threats to plants include attacking organisms, such as bacteria, viruses, fungi, or parasites (This is familiar territory as those are the same types of organisms that we humans also have to battle against.); environmental conditions, such as strong ultraviolet rays or reduced ultraviolet rays, a low level of oxygen, hot or cold temperatures, a too-salty environment and other threatening issues to the plant. Some organisms on and in the plant act as growth promoters for it or assist in making nutrients available to the plant or even help with reproduction. And just like humans, plants need enzymes and antioxidants, which are provided to the plants from the organisms that live in and on it.

Organisms in and on our body's help us fight off disease causing organisms, and this is also true in the plant world. It was a battle between the mold Penicillium and the bacterium Staphylococci that led to the development of the first man-made anti-biotic Penicillin. This points out two very important facts: 1) This battle between two types of organisms displays the competition that exists in nature between organisms, clearly the Penicillium mold won over the bacteria Staphylococci. 2) The course of medicine was forever changed, and humans benefitted from the victor in that fight.

Just as technology is allowing us to see the different organisms in and on us and how those relationships result in our health status, the same is happening in research on plants. Research is revealing that it is the organisms in and on the plants that produce the secondary metabolites which are biologically active and shape the health and life of the plant. These secondary metabolites also affect our bodies. It has been stated this way by numerous researchers: "Secondary metabolites are biologically active compounds that are an important source of anticancer, antioxidant, antidiabetic, immunosuppressive, antifungal, anti-oomycete, antibacterial, insecticidal, nematicidal, and antiviral agents."[419] [420] [421] [422] [423] [424] [425] [426] [427]

It's not just the pharmaceutical industry that is looking at how plants can be used to their advantage. The food industry too is researching the use of plants for their antioxidant abilities as well. The metabolites produced from organisms and plants have powerful antioxidants. The food industry has been and continues to research the use of plant antioxidants in processed foods to serve a number of functions. First, consumers have showed their concerns regarding synthetic ingredients and their preference for natural ingredients, consequentially the food industry is replacing various synthetic ingredients with natural antioxidants instead. Second, natural antioxidants are being used to hinder oxidation thereby extending shelf life. Third, plants are being used to enhance color, flavor and aroma of processed foods. If the billion-dollar food industry is looking at these strong anti-oxidants, doesn't it make sense for us to be consuming them daily in their natural forms, that being in vegetables and fruits, instead of processed foods?

Let's Sum This Up

Research studies are fascinating. In the plethora of research studies showing positive health benefits from a diet high in plants, most studies look at single plants, especially the older studies. But this is not the reality of how people eat. For example, some people love broccoli and may eat it once a week, or a person who drinks tea usually does so every day. But studies often look at just the one food they are studying and the other foods eaten are not taken into consideration at all, while they also affect the person's health. Take green tea; there are numerous studies on the health benefits of green tea, particularly from the compound EGCG (epigallocatechin gallate), which provides a number of health benefits, including the ability to keep blood glucose levels low. Yet, even though many studies can directly prove that the EGCG lowered blood glucose levels some of the studies point out that still more research is needed as certain people retain high glucose levels in spite of green tea consumption. This will happen if people are still eating sugar and carbohydrates that are driving their blood glucose levels up, and/or if these people are still eating inflammatory foods like dairy products and sugar, which both play a role in blocking the uptake of glucose due to the inflammation these foods produce.

On the other hand, all of the studies on vegetarians and Seventh Day Adventists' show only numerous health benefits without inconsistent results because these are people who consistently eat diets high in vegetables. And that consistent dietary factor is where the rubber meets the road; true results are seen in the human body when plants are consumed more than other foods.

There is no arguing that people with diets high in plants and low in sugar and processed foods do not have the incidence of hypertension, high cholesterol, type 2 diabetes, and metabolic syndrome that people eating the standard American diet (SAD) have. The overall diet is the determining factor. It is the total amount of phytonutrients consumed on a regular basis that creates the whole. This is referenced in the chapter titled "The Sum Is Greater Than the Parts," where it was discussed that the plants eaten are the substance that healthy bacteria and other organisms develop from. (A weird and amazing fact that makes you realize that much about our human body can easily be the material for Sci-Fi.)

Stated another way: The foods you eat are the soil for which organisms will develop from. Many studies have proven that healthy gut organisms are able to degrade and then extract the nutrients from food eaten. This is quite different from what unhealthy gut organisms do, as they do not pull out the healthy phytonutrients needed and they also store the calories as fat instead of utilizing them. Once someone eats healthfully, and mostly plant foods, they will alter their gut microbiota to the point that healthy organisms will be thriving in their intestines. Consequently, those healthier organisms are able to extract the nutrients your body needs. It takes healthy foods to create a healthy environment, and then that healthy environment pays it forward to your entire body by supplying it with more nutrients. The foods eaten dictate the organisms, which then dictate the health of your entire body. It is not one magical substance from fruits and vegetables; it is the whole array, as pointed out in the chapter "The Rainbow of Phytonutrients." The result from a diet of different and varied plants supplying the range of phytonutrients is a gut microbiota inhabited by diverse organisms. The diversification of organisms in your gut benefits your whole body, your overall health. It protects all your organs and systems and keeps your body functioning optimally.

The synergy that occurs between different phytonutrients in a shared environment is vitally important. Phytonutrients from previously eaten vegetables are the catalysts for action for subsequent phytonutrients consumed. In Chinese medicine, herbal formulas are created so that the effects of one or more herbs get potentiated by the other herbs in the formula. This is why specific herbs are chosen when creating herbal formulas. Chinese medicine is always about creating balance; in creating an herbal formula the synergism of the herbs brings that balance, not individual herbs. In the field of pharmacology this is called "potentization," the interaction between two or more drugs that creates a response that is greater than the response would have been from those drugs if used solely.

As discussed in the previous chapter "Plants Used as Pharmaceuticals," at the time of this writing there are over 200 patents in process to the FDA to make medications from plants. Even the billion-dollar food industry sees potential in using the powerful antioxidants from plants in processed foods. I believe you should eat the full plant, as you will get all the benefits that are there for you to be healthy. As stated earlier, your body does not fully utilize supplements. You are better off eating a diet high in plants to get the vitamins, minerals, and phytonutrients your body needs.

Humans, in our current form, have been in existence for only about 200,000 years. For about 199,900 of those years humans ate only foods that grew or could be caught, and they lived in better health than we do today. If for almost 200,000 years humans thrived on plants and some animal food sources don't you think your body would too? This is the perfect time to start questioning why you think you need any processed food at all?

This is the first time in human existence that humans have eaten millions of tons of sugar. This escalation in sugar consumption coincides directly with the increases in chronic health problems and especially autoimmune problems.

One last and crucial point: This is the first time in human existence that we are eating large volumes of processed foods. The results of this hundred-year "experiment" are not good. If you go back to a plant-based diet, like most humans had for most of our existence, you will see and feel enormous benefits.

What could possibly be the harm of giving up those comfort foods you repeatedly eat? For most people it is an emotional issue, because the reality is, it is not a physical need to eat processed foods. There is a need to eat, and if you eat just the foods that are natural, your body and brain will function at their best - the way they are supposed to.

It is very curious that most people will very readily pop a pill, a chemical that is not easily metabolized and usually creates harm, but most people will not make dietary changes to help themselves, even simple changes like increasing vegetable intake.

That is enough right? If that is not enough information to spur you to quickly changing your diet ... I don't know what would be!

Information is just simply information until it is applied. You now know that eating the vegetables listed in all their wide array of colors will improve your health. If you want better quality of life, the very first factor that can bestow better quality of life to you is your health. It is not hard to eat healthfully.

By eating mostly vegan you can:

- ❖ Have better brain function. Studies have shown that some phytonutrients and the short-chain fatty acids cross the brain-blood-barrier affecting the brain.
- ❖ Maintain a healthy blood pressure.
- ❖ Keep your cholesterol at a healthy level.
- ❖ Reduce your risk of getting diabetes.
- ❖ Lower your chances of getting metabolic syndrome.
- ❖ Reduce your risk of having a heart attack.
- ❖ Lower your chances of getting an autoimmune disease or, if you have an autoimmune disease,

eating vegan has been shown to reduce the symptoms and slow down its progress.
❖ Reduce your chances of developing a cancer. The American Cancer Society states in their 2014 Cancer Facts and Figures that the World Cancer Research Fund has estimated that "up to one-third of the cancer cases that occur in economically developed countries like the US are related to overweight or obesity, physical inactivity, and/or poor nutrition, and thus could also be prevented."[428] The best way to lose weight and maintain a healthy weight is by having a diet proportionally heavier in vegetables and fruits.
❖ Slow down the aging process.
❖ Feel better every day!

The all-important take-away is this: Eat several servings of vegetables every day and as many different ones as you can get and you will be healthy!

Chapter References

Important Points

[1] The American Journal of Clinical Nutrition, Poti JM, Mendez MA, Ng SW, et al. Is the Degree of Food Processing and Convenience Linked with the Nutritional Quality of Foods Purchased by US Households?, vol 101, no 6, Jun 2015, 1251-1262, doi.org/10.3945/ajcn.114.100925.

[2] The American Journal of Clinical Nutrition, Poti JM, Mendez MA, Ng SW, et al. Is the Degree of Food Processing and Convenience Linked with the Nutritional Quality of Foods Purchased by US Households?, vol 101, no 6, Jun 2015, 1251-1262, doi.org/10.3945/ajcn.114.100925.

[3] Journal of the American Medical Association, Micha R, Penalvo JL, Cudhea F, et al. Association Between Dietary Factors and Mortality From Heart Disease, Stroke, and Type 2 Diabetes in the United States, Mar 7, 2017, vol 317, no 9, 912-924, doi:10.1001/jama.2017.0947.

[4] Journal of the American Medical Association, Micha R, Penalvo JL, Cudhea F, et al. Association Between Dietary Factors and Mortality From Heart Disease, Stroke, and Type 2 Diabetes in the United States, Mar 7, 2017, vol 317, no 9, 912-924, doi:10.1001/jama.2017.0947.

Obesity Rates, Why we Have to Take a Look

[5] CDC, National Center for Health Statistics. (2020). Hales CM, Carroll MD, Fryar CD, et al. Prevalence of Obesity and Severe Obesity Among Adults: United States, 2017-2018, NCHS Data Brief No 360, Feb 2020, https://www.cdc.gov/nchs/products/databriefs/db360.htm.

[6] CDC, National Center for Health Statistics. (2020). Hales CM, Carroll MD, Fryar CD, et al. Prevalence of Obesity and Severe Obesity Among Adults: United States, 2017-2018, NCHS Data Brief No 360, Feb 2020, https://www.cdc.gov/nchs/products/databriefs/db360.htm.

[7] CDC, National Center for Health Statistics. (2020). Hales CM, Carroll MD, Fryar CD, et al. Prevalence of Obesity and Severe Obesity Among Adults: United States, 2017-2018, NCHS Data Brief No 360, Feb 2020, https://www.cdc.gov/nchs/products/databriefs/db360.htm.

[8] CDC, National Center for Health Statistics. (2020). Hales CM, Carroll MD, Fryar CD, et al. Prevalence of Obesity and Severe Obesity Among Adults: United States, 2017-2018, NCHS Data Brief No 360, Feb 2020, https://www.cdc.gov/nchs/products/databriefs/db360.htm.

[9] CDC, National Center for Health Statistics. (2020). Hales CM, Carroll MD, Fryar CD, et al. Prevalence of Obesity and Severe Obesity Among Adults: United States, 2017-2018, NCHS Data Brief No 360, Feb 2020, https://www.cdc.gov/nchs/products/databriefs/db360.htm.

[10] CDC, National Center for Health Statistics. (2020). Hales CM, Carroll MD, Fryar CD, et al. Prevalence of Obesity and Severe Obesity Among Adults: United States, 2017-2018, NCHS Data Brief No 360, Feb 2020, https://www.cdc.gov/nchs/products/databriefs/db360.htm.

[11] CDC, National Center for Health Statistics. (2020). Hales CM, Carroll MD, Fryar CD, et al. Prevalence of Obesity and Severe Obesity Among Adults: United States, 2017-2018, NCHS Data Brief No 360, Feb 2020, https://www.cdc.gov/nchs/products/databriefs/db360.htm.

[12] Gallup, Well Being, Reinhart RJ, More Americans Say They Weigh 200 Lbs. or More This Decade, Nov 27, 2019, https://news.gallup.com/poll/268847/americans-say-weigh-200-lbs-decade.aspx.

[13] Harvard School of Public Health, Department of Nutrition, Hasker RR, Food for Your Heart: Manual for Patient and Physician, New York: American Heart Association, 1952.

[14] Lancet, Infant and Adult Obesity (Editorial), Jan 5, 1974, 17-18, doi.org/10.1016/S0140-6736(74)93004-9.

[15] Lancet, Infant and Adult Obesity (Editorial), Jan 5, 1974, 17-18, doi.org/10.1016/S0140-6736(74)93004-9.

[16] Lancet, Infant and Adult Obesity (Editorial), Jan 5, 1974, 17-18, doi.org/10.1016/S0140-6736(74)93004-9.

[17] Lancet, Infant and Adult Obesity (Editorial), Jan 5, 1974, 17-18, doi.org/10.1016/S0140-6736(74)93004-9.

[18] Department of Health and Human Services (US), Promoting Health/Preventing Disease: Objectives for the Nation, Washington, 1980.

[19] Department of Health and Human Services (US), Healthy People 2000: National Health Promotion and and Disease Prevention Objectives, Washington, 1990.

[20] American Cancer Society. Cancer Facts & Figures 2017. Atlanta: American Cancer Society: 2017. source www.iarc.fr.

[21] Gallup, Well Being, Reinhart RJ, More Americans Say They Weigh 200 Lbs. or More This Decade, Nov 27, 2019, https://news.gallup.com/poll/268847/americans-say-weigh-200-lbs-decade.aspx.

[22] Gallup, Well Being, Reinhart RJ, More Americans Say They Weigh 200 Lbs. or More This Decade, Nov 27, 2019, https://news.gallup.com/poll/268847/americans-say-weigh-200-lbs-decade.aspx.

[23] CDC, National Center for Health Statistics. (2010). Ogden CL, Carroll MD, Prevalence of Overweight, Obesity, and Extreme Obesity Among Adults: United States, Trends1960-1962 Through2007-2008, National Health and Nutrition Examination Survey, Jun 2010, https://www.cdc.gov/nchs/data/hestat/obesity_adult_07_08/obesity_adult_07_08.pdf .

[24] Lancet Body-mass Index and all-Cause Mortality: Individual-Participant-Data Meta-Analysis of 239 Prospective Studies in Four Continents, July 13, 106, vol 388, issue 10046, p 776-786. doi:10.1016/S0140-6736(16)30175-1.

Your Microbiome: What It Is, What Influences It, & Why It Matters

[25] Gut from the British medical Journal, The Gut Microbiota and Host Health: a new Clinical Frontier, Marchesi J, Adams D, Fava F, et al. February 2016, vol 65, no 2, 330-339, doi:10.1136/gutjnl-2015-309990.

[26] Science Magazine by the American Association for the Advancement of Science, Muegge B, Kuczynski J, Knights D, et al. Diet Drives Convergence in gut Microbiome Functions Across Mammalian Phylogeny and Within Humans, March 14, 2012, vol 332, no 6032, 970-974, doi:10.1126/science.1198719.

[27] Science Magazine by the American Association for the Advancement of Science, Muegge B, Kuczynski J, Knights D, et al. Diet Drives Convergence in gut Microbiome Functions Across Mammalian Phylogeny and Within Humans,

March 14, 2012, vol 332, no 6032, 970-974, doi:10.1126/science.1198719.
[28] Science Magazine by the American Association for the Advancement of Science, Muegge B, Kuczynski J, Knights D, et al. Diet Drives Convergence in gut Microbiome Functions Across Mammalian Phylogeny and Within Humans, March 14, 2012, vol 332, no 6032, 970-974, doi:10.1126/science.1198719.

How Do I Get Calcium?

[29] Vitamin and Mineral Requirements in Human Nutrition Second Edition, World Health Organization and Food and Agricultural Organization of the United Nations, 2004, https://apps.who.int/iris/bitstream/handle/10665/42716/9241546123.pdf
[30] Nature Reviews. Endocrinology, Cauly JA, Chalhoub D, Kassem AM, et al. Geographic and Ethnic Disparities in Osteoporotic Fractures, June 2014, vol 10 no 6, 338-351, doi:10.1038/nrendo.2014.51.
[31] Journal of Bone and Mineral Research, Yang S, Feskanich D, Willett WC, et al. Association Between Global Biomarkers of Oxidative Stress and hip Fracture in Postmenopausal Women: a Prospective Study, December 2014, vol 29 no 12, 2577-2583, doi:10.1002/jbmr.2302.
[32] Nature Reviews. Endocrinology, Cauly JA, Chalhoub D, Kassem AM, et al. Geographic and Ethnic Disparities in Osteoporotic Fractures, June 2014, vol 10 no 6, 338-351, doi:10.1038/nrendo.2014.51.
[33] The Nurses' Health Study Annual Newsletter, Dr. Colditz G, Dr. Willett W, Dr. Feskanich D, vol 11, 2004, https://www.nurseshealthstudy.org/sites/default/files/pdfs/n2004.pdf
[34] Osteoporosis International, Knapen MH, Schurgers LJ, Vermeer C, Vitamin K2 Supplementation Improves hip Bone Geometry and Strength Indices in Postmenopausal Women, July 2007, vol 18 no 7, 963-972, doi:10.1007/s00198-007-0337-9.
[35] Public Health Nutrition, Thorpe L, Knulsen S, Beeson W, et al. Effects of Meat Consumption and Vegetarian Diet on Risk of Wrist Fracture Over 25 Years in a cohort of Peri- and Postmenopausal Women, June 2008. Vol 11, no 6, 564-572, doi:10.1017/S1368980007000808.
[36] Public Health Nutrition, Thorpe L, Knulsen S, Beeson W, et al. Effects of Meat Consumption and Vegetarian Diet on Risk of Wrist Fracture Over 25 Years in a cohort of Peri- and Postmenopausal Women, June 2008. Vol 11, no 6, 564-572, doi:10.1017/S1368980007000808.
[37] European Journal of Drug Metabolism and Pharmacokinetics, Vitale DC, Piazza C, Melilli B, et al. Isoflavones: Estrogenic Activity, Biological Effect and Bioavailability, March 2013, vol 38, no 1, 15-25, doi:10.1007/s13318-012-0112-y.

How Do I Get Protein?

[38] Metabolism: clinical and experimental, Jenkins DJ, Kendall CW, Faulkner D, et al. A Dietary Portfolio Approach to Cholesterol Reduction: Combined Effects of Plant Sterols, Vegetable Proteins, and Viscous Fibers in Hypercholesterolemia, December 2002, vol 51, no 12, 1596-1604, doi:10.1053/meta.2002.35578.
[39] Metabolism: clinical and experimental, Jenkins DJ, Kendall CW, Faulkner D, et al. A Dietary Portfolio Approach to Cholesterol Reduction: Combined Effects of Plant Sterols, Vegetable Proteins, and Viscous Fibers in Hypercholesterolemia, December 2002, vol 51, no 12, 1596-1604, doi:10.1053/meta.2002.35578.
[40] Nutrition and Cancer, Kim MK, Kim JH, Nam SJ, et al. Dietary Intake of Soy

Protein and Tofu in Association with Breast Cancer Risk Based on a Case-Control Study, 2008, vol 60, no 5, 568-576, doi:10.1080/01635580801966203.

Getting Enough Other Vital Nutrients
[41] National Institutes of Health, Office of Dietary Supplements.
[42] Nature, Wang Z, Klipfell E, Bennett BJ, et al. Gut Flora Metabolism of Phosphatidlycholine Promotes Cardiovascular Disease, April 7, 2011, vol 472, no 7341, 57-63, doi:10.1038/nature09922.

Why This Is a Healthy Way to Eat
[43] The BMJ, Tong TYN, Appleby PN, Bradbury KE, et al. Risks of Ischaemic Heart Disease and Stroke in Meat Eaters, Fish Eaters, and Vegetarians Over 18 Years of Follow-up: Results From the Prospective EPIC-Oxford Study, September 4, 2019, vol 366, 14,897, doi:10.1136/bmj.14897.
[44] The BMJ, Tong TYN, Appleby PN, Bradbury KE, et al. Risks of Ischaemic Heart Disease and Stroke in Meat Eaters, Fish Eaters, and Vegetarians Over 18 Years of Follow-up: Results From the Prospective EPIC-Oxford Study, September 4, 2019, vol 366, 14,897, doi:10.1136/bmj.14897.
[45] Nutrients, Glick-Bauer M, Yeh MC, The Health Advantage of a Vegan Diet: Exploring the Gut Microbiota Connection, November 2014, vol 6, no 11, 4822-4838, doi:10.3390/nu6114822.
[46] Health Day News, Goodman B, Health Day Reporter, Vegetarian Diet May Help Lower Blood Pressure, Feb 24, 2014.
[47] The American Journal of Clinical Nutrition, Winston C, Health Effects of Vegan Diets, March 11, 2009, vol 89, no 5, 1627S-1633S. doi.org/10.3945.
[48] Journal of the American Medical Association, Gardner, C D Phd, Trepanowski J F, PhD, Del Gobbo L C Phd, et al. Effect of Low-Fat vs Low-Carbohydrate Diet on 12-Month Weight Loss on Over Weight Adults and the Association with Genotype Pattern or Insulin Secretion, Feb 20, 2018, 319(7):667-679, doi:10.1001/jama.2018.0245.
[49] European Journal of Epidemiology, Commenges D, Scotet V, Renaud, et al. Intake of flavonoids and risk of dementia. 2000;16:357–363, doi:10.1023/A:1007614613771.
[50] American Journal of Epidemiology, Letenneur L, Proust-Lima C, Le Gouge A, Flavonoid Intake and Cognitive Decline Over a 10-Year Period, Jun 15, 2007, 15;165(12):1364-71, doi:10:193/aje/kwm036.
[51] American Journal of Epidemiology, Letenneur L, Proust-Lima C, Le Gouge A, Flavonoid Intake and Cognitive Decline Over a 10-Year Period, Jun 15, 2007, 15;165(12):1364-71, doi:10:193/aje/kwm036

How Do You Want to Age? Your Lifestyle Effects How You Age
[52] Complementary Therapies in Medicine, Sutliffe JT, Wilson LD, de Heer HD, et al. C-Reactive Protein Response to a Vegan Lifestyle Intervention, Feb 23, 2015, vol 1: 32-7, doi: 10.1016/j.ctm.2014.11.001.
[53] Nutrients, Glick-Bauer M, Yeh MC, The Health Advantage of a Vegan Diet, Oct 31, 2014, vol 6, no 11, 4822-4838, doi:10.3390/nu6114822.
[54] Nutrients, Glick-Bauer M, Yeh MC, The Health Advantage of a Vegan Diet, Oct 31, 2014, vol 6, no 11, 4822-4838, doi:10.3390/nu6114822.

Foods Affect the Microbiome

[55] Journal of Clinical Gastroenterology, Szaleczky E, Pronai L, Nakazawa H, et al. Evidence of in vivo Peroxynitrite Formation in Patients with Colorectal Carcinoma, Higher Plasma nitrate/nitrite Levels, and Lower Protection Against Oxygen Free Radicals, January 2000, vol 30, no 1, 47-51, PMID 10636209.

[56] Gut, Kimura H, Hokari R, Miura S, et al. Increased Expression of an Inducible Isoform on Nitric Oxide Synthase and the Formation of Peroxynitrite in Colonic Mucosa of Patients with Active Ulcerative Colitis, February 1998, vol 42, no 2, 180-187, doi:10.1136/gut.42.2.180.

[57] Free Radical Research, Whiteman M, Halliwell B, Protection Against Peroxynitrite-Dependent Tyrosine Nitration and Alpha 1-Antiprtoeinase Inactivation by Ascorbic Acid. A Comparison with other Biological Antioxidants, September 1996, vol 25, no 3, 275-283, PMID:8889493.

[58] Proceeding of the National Academy of Sciences of the United States of America, Hooper DC, Spitsin S, Kean RB, et al. Uric Acid a Natural Scavenger of Peroxynitrite, in Experimental Allergic Encephalomyelitis and Multiple Sclerosis, January 20, 1998, vol 95, no 2, 675-680, doi:10.1073/pnas.95.2.675.

[59] Phytotherapy Research, Choi Js, Chung HY, Kang SS, et al. The Structure-Activity Relationship of Flavonoids as Scavengers of Peroxynitrite, May 2002, vol 16, no 3, 232-235, doi:10.1002/ptr.828.

[60] Toxicology in vitro: an International Journal Published in Association with BIBRA, Heijnen CG, Haenen GR, van Acker FA, et al. Flavonoids as Peroxynitrite Scavengers: the Role of the Hydroxyl Groups, February 2001, vol 15, no 1, 3-6, PMID:11256893.

[61] Phytochemistry, Harborne JB, Williams CA, Advances in Flavonoid Research Since 1992, November 200, vol 55, no 6, 481-504, PMID:11130659.

[62] American Journal of Clinical Nutrition, Nijveldt RJ, van Nood E, van Hoorn DE, et al. Flavonoids: a Review of Probable Mechanisms o Action and Potential Applications, October 2001, vol 74, no 4, 418-425, doi:10.1093/ajcn/74.4.418.

[63] World Journal of Gastroenterology, Rose P, Nam Ong C, Whiteman M, Protective Effects of Asian Green Vegetables Against Oxidant Induced Cytotoxicity, December 28, 2005, vol 11, no 48, 7607-7614, doi:10.3748/wjg.v11.j48.7607.

[64] Nature Medicine, Hazen S, Koeth R, Zeneng W, et al. Intestinal Microbiota Metabolism of L-Carnitine, a Nutrient in red Meat, Promotes Atherosclerosis, April 7, 2013, vol 19, 576-585.

[65] Nature Medicine, Hazen S, Koeth R, Zeneng W, et al. Intestinal Microbiota Metabolism of L-Carnitine, a Nutrient in red Meat, Promotes Atherosclerosis, April 7, 2013, vol 19, 576-585.

[66] Nature Medicine, Hazen S, Koeth R, Zeneng W, et al. Intestinal Microbiota Metabolism of L-Carnitine, a Nutrient in red Meat, Promotes Atherosclerosis, April 7, 2013, vol 19, 576-585.

[67] Nature Medicine, Hazen S, Koeth R, Zeneng W, et al. Intestinal Microbiota Metabolism of L-Carnitine, a Nutrient in red Meat, Promotes Atherosclerosis, April 7, 2013, vol 19, 576-585.

[68] Science, Wu GD, Chen J, Hoffman C, et al. Linking Long-Term Dietary Patterns with Gut Microbial Enterotypes, October 7, 2011, vol 334, no 6052, 105-108, doi:10.1126/science.1208344.

[69] Science, Wu GD, Chen J, Hoffman C, et al. Linking Long-Term Dietary Patterns with Gut Microbial Enterotypes, October 7, 2011, vol 334, no 6052,

105-108, doi:10.1126/science.1208344.

[70] Proceedings of the National Academy of Sciences of the United States of America, De Filippo C, Cavalieri D, Di Paola M, et al. Impact of Diet in Shaping gut Microbiota Revealed by a Comparative Study in Children from Europe and Rural Africa, August 17, 2010, vol 107, no 33, 14691-14696, doi:10.1073/pnas.1005963107.

[71] Nature, Ley PE, Turnbaugh PJ, Klein S, et al. Microbial Ecology: Human Gut Microbes Associated with Obesity, December 21, 2006, vol 444, no 7122, 1022-1023, doi:10.1038/4441022a.

[72] The American Journal of Clinical Nutrition, van Faassen A, Bol J, van Dokkum W, et al. Bile Acids, Neutral Steroids, and Bacteria in Feces as Affected by a Mixed, a Lacto-ovovegetraian and a Vegan Diet, December 1987, vol 46, no 6, 962-967, doi:10.1093/ajcn/46.6.962.

[73] Nutrients, Glick-Bauer M, Yeh MC, The Health Advantage of a Vegan Diet: Exploring the Gut Microbiota Connection, November 2014, vol 6, no 11, 4822-4838, doi:10.3390/nu6114822.

[74] British Journal of Nutrition, Benus RF, van der Werf TS, Weilling GW, Association Between Faecalibacterium prausntzii and Dietary Fibre in Colonic Fermentation in Healthy Human Subjects, September 2010, vol 104, no 5, 693-700, doi:10.1017/S0007114510001030.

[75] BMC Systems Biology, Henson M, Phalak P, Microbiota Dysbiosis in Inflammatory Bowel Diseases: in silico Investigation of the Oxygen Hypothesis, December 28, 2017, vol 11, 145, doi:10.1186/s12918-017-0522-1.

[76] Science magazine by the American Association for the Advancement of Science, Muegge B, Kuczynski J, Knights D, Diet Drives Convergence in gut Microbiome Functions Across Mammalian Phylogeny and Within Humans, May 20, 2011, vol 332, no 6032, 970-974, doi:10.1126/science.1198719.

The Western Diet's Influence on the Microbiome

[77] Journal of the American Medical Association, Mokdad AH, Marks JS, Stroup DF, et al. Actual Causes of Death in the United States, 2000, Mar 10, 2004, vol 291, no 10, 1238-1245, doi:10.1001/jama.291.10.1238.

[78] Journal of the American Medical Association, Mokdad AH, Marks JS, Stroup DF, et al. Actual Causes of Death in the United States, 2000, Mar 10, 2004, vol 291, no 10, 1238-1245, doi:10.1001/jama.291.10.1238.

[79] Journal of the American Medical Association, Murray C JL, Abraham J, Ali M K, US Burden of Disease Collaborators et al. The State of US Health, 1990-2010, Burden of Diseases, Injuries, and Risk Factors, Aug 14, 2013, vol 310, no 6, 591-606, doi:10.1001/jama.2013.13805.

[80] Journal of the American Medical Association, Murray C JL, Abraham J, Ali M K, US Burden of Disease Collaborators et al. The State of US Health, 1990-2010, Burden of Diseases, Injuries, and Risk Factors, Aug 14, 2013, vol 310, no 6, 591-606, doi:10.1001/jama.2013.13805.

[81] Journal of the American Medical Association, Murray C JL, Abraham J, Ali M K, US Burden of Disease Collaborators et al. The State of US Health, 1990-2010, Burden of Diseases, Injuries, and Risk Factors, Aug 14, 2013, vol 310, no 6, 591-606, doi:10.1001/jama.2013.13805.

[82] Journal of Royal Society Medicine, Pallister T, Spector TD, Food: a new Form of Personalized (gut Microbiome) medicine for chronic diseases?, Sep 2016, 109(9):331-336. doi:10.1177/0141076816658786.

[83] Current Gastroenterology Reports, Shivashankar R, Lewis JD, The Role of Diet in Inflammatory Bowel Disease, May 2017, vol 19, no 5, 22,

doi:10.1007/s11894-017-0563-z.
[84] Nature, Gewirtz A. Chassaing B, Koren O, et al. Dietary Emulsifiers Impact the Mouse Gut Microbiota Promoting Colitis and Metabolic Syndrome, March 5, 2015, 519(7541)):92-96, doi: 10.1038/nature1423.2.
[85] Nature, Gewirtz A. Chassaing B, Koren O, et al. Dietary Emulsifiers Impact the Mouse Gut Microbiota Promoting Colitis and Metabolic Syndrome, March 5, 2015, 519(7541)):92-96, doi: 10.1038/nature1423.2.
[86] Cancer Research, Viennois E, Gewirtz, A, Merlin D, et al. Dietary Emulsifier-Induced Low-Grade Inflammation Promotes Colon Carcinogenesis, January 1 2017, vol 77, no 1, 27-40, doi:10.1158/0008-5472.CAN-16-1359.
[87] Gut, Roberts CL, Keita AV, Duncan SH, O'Kennedy N, et al. Translocation of Crohn's Disease Escherichia coli Across M-Cells: Contrasting Effects of Soluble Plant Fibres and Emulsifiers, October 2010, vol 59, no 10, 1331-1339, doi:10.1136/gut.2009.195370.
[88] Journal of Crohn's & colitis, Roberts CL, Rushworth SL, Richman E, et al. Hypothesis: Increased Consumption of Emulsifiers as an Explanation for the Rising incidence of Crohn's Disease, May 2013, vol 7, no 4, 338-341, doi:10.1016/j.crohns.2013.01.004
[89] Gut, Chassaing B, Van de Wiele T, De Bodt J, et al. Dietary Emulsifiers Directly Alter Human Microbiota Composition and Gene Expression ex vivo Potentiating Intestinal Inflammation, August 2017, vol 66, no 8,1414-1427, doi:10.1136/gutjnl-2016-313099.
[90] Gut Microbes, Suez J, Korem T, Zilberman-Schapira G, et al. Non-Caloric Artificial Sweeteners and the Microbiome: Findings and Challenges, April 1 2015, 6(2):149-155, doi: 10.1080/19490976.2015.1017700..
[91] Gut Microbes, Suez J, Korem T, Zilberman-Schapira G, et al. Non-Caloric Artificial Sweeteners and the Microbiome: Findings and Challenges, April 1 2015, 6(2):149-155, doi:10.1080/19490976.2015.1017700.
[92] Gut Microbes, Suez J, Korem T, Zilberman-Schapira G, et al. Non-Caloric Artificial Sweeteners and the Microbiome: Findings and Challenges, April 1 2015, 6(2):149-155, doi:10.1080/19490976.2015.1017700.
[93] Gut Microbes, Suez J, Korem T, Zilberman-Schapira G, et al. Non-Caloric Artificial Sweeteners and the Microbiome: Findings and Challenges, April 1 2015, 6(2):149-155, doi:10.1080/19490976.2015.1017700.
[94] Obesity (Silver Spring, Md), Fowler SP, Williams K, Resendaz RG, et al. Fueling the Obesity Epidemic? Artificially Sweetened Beverage use and Long-Term Weight Gain, August 2008, vol 16, no 8, 1894-1900, doi:10.1038/oby.2008.284.
[95] Behavioral Brain Research, Swithers SF, Laboy AF, Clark K, et al. Experience with the High-Intensity Sweetener Saccharin Impairs Glucose Homeostasis and GLP-1 Release in rats, July 15, 2012, vol 233, no 1, 1-14, doi:10.1016/j.bbr.2012.04.024.
[96] Behavioral Brain Research, Swithers SF, Laboy AF, Clark K, et al. Experience with the High-Intensity Sweetener Saccharin Impairs Glucose Homeostasis and GLP-1 Release in rats, July 15, 2012, vol 233, no 1, 1-14, doi:10.1016/j.bbr.2012.04.024.
[97] Journal of General Internal Medicine, Gardener H, Rundek T, Markert M, et al. Diet Soft Drink Consumption is Associated with an Increased Risk of Vascular Events in the Northern Manhattan Study, September 2012, vol 27, no 9, 1120-1126, doi:10.1007/s11606=011-968-2
[98] Gut, Cani PD, Human gut Microbiome: Hopes, Threats and Promises, September 2018, vol 67, no 9, 1716-1725, doi:10.1136/gutjnl-2018-316723.
[99] Gut, Cani PD, Human gut Microbiome: Hopes, Threats and Promises, September 2018, vol 67, no 9, 1716-1725, doi:10.1136/gutjnl-2018-316723.

[100] Nutrients, Mills S, Stanton C, Lane JA, et al. Precision Nutrition and the Microbiome, Part I: Current State of the Science, April 2019, vol 11, no 4, 923, doi"10.3390/nu11040923.

Modern Research Reveals

[101] The ISME Journal, Walker AW, Ince J, Duncan SH, et al. Dominant and Diet-responsive Groups of Bacteria Within the Human Colonic Microbiota, February 2011, vol 5, no 2, 220-230, doi:10.1038/ismej.2010.118.
[102] Gut, Cani PD, Human gut Microbiome: Hopes, Threats and Promises, September 2018, vol 67, no 9, 1716-1725, doi:10.1136/gutjnl-2018-316723.
[103] Nutrients, Klimenko NS, Tyakht AV, Popenko AS, et al. Microbiome Responses to an Uncontrolled Short-Term Diet Intervention in the Frame of the Citizen Science ProjectMay 2018, vol 10, no 5, 576, doi:10.3390/nu10050576.
[104] Science magazine by the American Association for the Advancement of Science, Muegge B, Kuczynski J, Knights D, Diet Drives Convergence in gut Microbiome Functions Across Mammalian Phylogeny and Within Humans, May 20, 2011, vol 332, no 6032, 970-974, doi:10.1126/science.1198719.
[105] Nature, Turnbaugh PJ, David LA, Maurice CF, et al. Diet Rapidly and Reproducibly Alters the Human gut Microbiome, January 23, 2014, vol 505, no 7484, 559-563, doi:10.1038/nature12820.
[106] Nature, Turnbaugh PJ, David LA, Maurice CF, et al. Diet Rapidly and Reproducibly Alters the Human gut Microbiome, January 23, 2014, vol 505, no 7484, 559-563, doi:10.1038/nature12820.
[107] Nature, Turnbaugh PJ, David LA, Maurice CF, et al. Diet Rapidly and Reproducibly Alters the Human gut Microbiome, January 23, 2014, vol 505, no 7484, 559-563, doi:10.1038/nature12820.
[108] Nature, Yoshimoto S, Loo TM, Atarashi K, et al. Obesity- Induced gut Microbial Metabolite Promotes Liver Cancer Through Senescence Sercretome, July 4, 2013, vol 499,no 7456, 97-101, doi:10.1038/nature12347.
[109] Nature, Turnbaugh PJ, David LA, Maurice CF, et al. Diet Rapidly and Reproducibly Alters the Human gut Microbiome, January 23, 2014, vol 505, no 7484, 559-563, doi:10.1038/nature12820.
[110] Nature Communications, O'Keefe, Li JV, Lahti L, et al. Fat, Fibre and Cancer Risk in African Americans and Rural Africans, April 28, 2015, vol 6, 6342, doi:10.1038/ncomms7342.

Research Links Western Diet to Health Problems

[111] International Journal of Obesity, Lee J, Pilli S, Gebremariam A, et al. Getting Heavier, Younger: Trajectories of Obesity Over the Life Course, April 2012, vol 34 no, 4, 614-623, doi:10.1038/ijo.2009.235.
[112] Complementary Therapies in Medicine, Sutliffe JT, Wilson LD, de Heer HD, et al. C-Reactive Protein Response to a Vegan Lifestyle Intervention. February 2015, vol 23, no 1, 32-37, doi:10.1016/j.ctim.2014.11.001
[113] Complementary Therapies in Medicine, Sutliffe JT, Wilson LD, de Heer HD, et al. C-Reactive Protein Response to a Vegan Lifestyle Intervention. February 2015, vol 23, no 1, 32-37, doi:10.1016/j.ctim.2014.11.001
[114] Cell, Clemente JC, Ursell LK, Parfrey LW, et al. The Impact of the gut Microbiota on Human Health: an Integrative View, March 16, 2012, vol 148, no, 6, 1258-1270, doi:10.1016/j.cell2012.01.035.
[115] Nature Reviews Immunology, Round JL, Mazmanian SK, The gut Microbiota Shapes Intestinal Immune Responses During Health and Disease, May 2009.

Vol 9, no 5, 313-323, doi:10.1038/nri2515

[116] Advances in Immunology, Chow J, Lee S, Shen Y, et al. Host-Bacterial Symbiosis in Health and Disease, August 8, 2011, vol 107, 243-274, doi:10.1016/B978-0-12-3813000-8.00008-3.

[117] Frontiers in Immunology, Statovci D, Aguilera M, MacSharry J, et al. The Impact of Western Diet and Nutrients on the Microbiota and Immune Responses at Mucosal Interfaces, July 28, 2017, vol 8, 838, doi:10.3389/fimmu.2017.00838.

[118] Trends in Immunology, Berbers RM, Nierkins S, van Larr JM, et al. Microbial Dysbiosis in Common Variable Immune Deficiences: Evidence, Causes, and Consequences, March 2017, vol 38, no 3, 206-216, doi:10.1016/j.it.2016.11.008.

[119] Diabetes, Alkanani A, Hara N, Gottlieb P, et al. Alterations in Intestinal Microbiota Correlates with Susceptibility to Type 1 Diabetes, October 2015, vol 64, no 10, 3510-3520, doi:10.2337/db14-1847.

[120] PLoS One, Miyake S, Kim S, Suda W, et al. Dysbiosis in the gut Microbiota of Patients with Multiple Sclerosis, with a Striking Depletion of Species Belonging to Clostridia XIVa and IV Clusters, September 14, 2015, vol 10, no 9, e0137429, doi:10.1371/journal.pone.0137429.

[121] Frontiers in Microbiology, Opazo MC, Ortega-Rocha EM, Coronado-Arrazola I, et al. Intestinal Microbiota Influences Non-intestinal Related Autoimmune Diseases, March 12, 2018, vol 9, 432, doi:10.3389/fmicb.2018.00432.

[122] Frontiers in Microbiology, Opazo MC, Ortega-Rocha EM, Coronado-Arrazola I, et al. Intestinal Microbiota Influences Non-intestinal Related Autoimmune Diseases, March 12, 2018, vol 9, 432, doi:10.3389/fmicb.2018.00432.

[123] The BMJ, Valdes A, Walter J, Segal E, et al. Role of the gut Microbiota in Nutrition and Health, June 13, 2018, doi:10.1136/bmj.k2179.

[124] Gut, Manichanh C, Rigottier-Gois L, Bonnaud E, et al. Reduced Diversity of Faecal Microbiota in Crohn's Disease Revealed by a Metagenomic Approach, February 2006, vol 55, no 2, 205-211, doi:10.1136/gut.2005.073817.

[125] The Journal of Allergy and Clinical Immunology, Wang M, Karlsson C, Olsson C, et al. Reduced Diversity in the Early Fecal Microbiota of Infants with Atopic Eczema, January 2008, vol 121, no 1, 129-134, doi:10.1016/j.jaci.2007.09.011.

[126] Diabetes, de Goffau M, Luopajarvi K, Knip M, et al. Fecal Microbiota Composition Differs Between Children with B-Cell Autoimmunity and Those Without, April 2013, vol 62, no 4, 1238-1244, doi:10.2337/db12-0526.

[127] Journal of Diabetes and Obesity, Lambeth S, Carson T, Lowe J, et al. Composition, Diversity and Abundance of Gut Microbiome in Prediabetes and Type 2 Diabetes, December 26, 2015, vol 2, no 3, 1-7, doi:10.15436/2376-0949.15.031.

[128] Arthritis & Rheumatology, Scher J, Ubeda C, Artacho A, et al. Decreased Bacterial Diversity Characterizes an Altered Gut Microbiota in Psoriatic Arthritis and Resembles Dysbiosis of Inflammatory Bowel Disease, January 2015, vol 67, no 1, 128-139, doi:10.1002/art.38892.

[129] European Heart Journal, Menni C, Lin C, Cecelja M, et al. Gut Microbial Diversity is Associated with Lower Arterial Stiffness in Women, July 1, 2018, vol 39, no 25, 2390-2397, doi:10.1093.eurheartj/ehy226.

[130] Nature, Turnbaugh PJ, Hamady M, Yatsunenko T, et al. A Core gut Microbiome in Obese and Lean Twins, January 22, 2009, vol 457, no 7228, 480-484, doi:10.1038/nature07540.

[131] Inflammation & Allergy - Drug Targets, Actis GC, The gut Microbiome, 2014, vol 13, no 4, 217-223, doi:10.2174/1871528113666140623113221.

[132] Annals of Rheumatic Diseases, Breban M, Tap J, Lebiome A, et al. Faecal

Microbiota Study Reveals Specific Dysbiosis in Spondyloarthritis, September 2017, vol 76, no 9, 1614-1622, doi:10.1136/annrheumdis-2016-211064.

[133] Annals of Rheumatic Diseases, Breban M, Tap J, Lebiome A, et al. Faecal Microbiota Study Reveals Specific Dysbiosis in Spondyloarthritis, September 2017, vol 76, no 9, 1614-1622, doi:10.1136/annrheumdis-2016-211064.

[134] Journal of Rheumatology, Vaahtovuo J, Munukka E, Korkeamäki M, et al. Fecal Microbiota in Early Rheumatoid Arthritis, August 2008, vol 35, no 8, 1500-1505, PMID:18528968.

[135] International Journal of Rheumatic Diseases, Sandhya P, Danda D, Sharma D, et al. Does the buck stop with the bugs?: An overview of microbial dysbiosis in rheumatoid arthritis, January 2016, vol19, no1, 8–20. doi: 10.1111/1756-185X.12728.

[136] Immunity, Wu HJ, Ivanov II, Darce J, et al. Gut-residing segmented filamentous bacteria drive autoimmune arthritis via T helper 17 cells, June 25; 2010, vol 32, no6, 815-27, doi:10.1016/j.immuni.2010.06.001.

[137] Nature, Ley RE, Turnbaugh PJ, Klein S, Microbial ecology: human gut microbes associated with Obesity, December 21, 2006, vol 444, no 7122, 1022-1023, doi:10.1038/4441022a.

[138] Nature, Turnbaugh PJ, Ley RE, Mahowald MA, et al. An Obesity-associated gut Microbiome with Increased Capacity for Energy Harvest, December 21, 2006, vol 444, no 7122, 1027-3101, doi:10.1038/nature05414.

[139] Nature, Turnbaugh PJ, Ley RE, Mahowald MA, et al. An Obesity-associated gut Microbiome with Increased Capacity for Energy Harvest, December 21, 2006, vol 444, no 7122, 1027-3101, doi:10.1038/nature05414.

[140] Nature, Turnbaugh PJ, Hamady M, Yatsunenko T, et al. A Core gut Microbiome in Obese and Lean Twins, January 22, 2009, vol 457, no 7228, 480-484, doi:10.10.38/nature07540.

[141] Gut, Dao MC, Everard A, Aron-Wisenewsky J, et al. Akkermansia Muciniphila and Improved Metabolic Health During a Dietary Intervention un Obesity: Relationshipwith gut Microbiome Richness and Ecology, March 2016, vol 65, no 3, 426-436, doi:10.1136/gutjnl-2014-308778.

[142] Nutrition & Diabetes, Fernandes J, Su W, Rahat-Rozenbloom S, et al. Adiposity, gut Microbiota and Faecal Short-chain fatty acids are Linked in Adult Humans, June 2014,vol 4, no 6, e121, doi:10.1038.nutd.2014.23.

[143] Proceedings of the National Academy of Sciences of the United States of America, De Filippo C, Cavalieri D, Di Paola M, et al. Impact of Diet in Shaping gut Microbiota Revealed by a Comparative Study in Children from Europe and Rural Africa, August 17, 2010, vol 107, no 33, 14691-14696, doi:10.1073/pnas.1005963107.

[144] Proceedings of the National Academy of Sciences of the United States of America, De Filippo C, Cavalieri D, Di Paola M, et al. Impact of Diet in Shaping gut Microbiota Revealed by a Comparative Study in Children from Europe and Rural Africa, August 17, 2010, vol 107, no 33, 14691-14696, doi:10.1073/pnas.1005963107.

[145] Frontiers in Physiology, Fransisco V, Pino J, Campos-Cabaleiro V, et al. Obesity, Fat Mass and Immune System: Role for Leptin, June 1, 2018, doi:10.3389/fphys.2018;9:640.

[146] Frontiers in Immunology, Statovci D, Aguilera M, MacSharry J, et al. The Impact of Western Diet and Nutrients on the Microbiota and Immune Responses at Mucosal Interfaces, July 28, 2017, vol 8, 838, doi:10.3389/fimmu.2017.00838.

[147] European Review for Medical and Pharmacological Sciences, Purchiaroni F, Tortora A, Gabrielli M, et al. The Role of Intestinal Microbiota and the Immune

System, February 2013, vol 17, no 3, 323-333, doi:10.3389/fimmu.2017.00838.

[148] Frontiers in Physiology, Fransisco V, Pino J, Campos-Cabaleiro V, et al. Obesity, Fat Mass and Immune System: Role for Leptin, June 1, 2018, doi:10.3389/fphys.2018;9:640.

[149] Frontiers in Physiology, Fransisco V, Pino J, Campos-Cabaleiro V, et al. Obesity, Fat Mass and Immune System: Role for Leptin, June 1, 2018, doi:10.3389/fphys.2018;9:640.

[150] Frontiers in Physiology, Fransisco V, Pino J, Campos-Cabaleiro V, et al. Obesity, Fat Mass and Immune System: Role for Leptin, June 1, 2018, doi:10.3389/fphys.2018;9:640.

[151] The Journal of Clinical Endocrinology and Metabolism, le Roux CW, Patterson M, Vincent RP, et al. Postprandial Plasma Ghrelin is Suppressed Proportional to Meal Calorie Content in normal-weight but not Obese Subjects, February 2005, vol 90, no 2, 1068-1071, doi:10.1210/jc.2004-1216.

[152] Asia Pacific Journal of Clinical Nutrition, Andarini S, Kangsaputra FB, Handayani D, Pre- and Postprandial Acylated Ghrelin in Obese and Normal Weight men, June 2017, vol 26, supp 1, S85-S91, doi:10.6133/apjcn.062017.s5.

[153] Nature, Turnbaugh PJ, David LA, Maurice CF, et al. Diet Rapidly and Reproducibly Alters the Human gut Microbiome, January 23, 2014, vol 505, no 7484, 559-563, doi:10.1038/nature12820.

Plant Foods Increase Bacterial Diversity

[154] Cell, Clemente JC, Ursell LK, Wegener Parfrey L, et al. The Impact of the gut Microbiota on Human Health: An Integrative View, March 16, 2012, vol 143, no 6, 1258-1270, doi:10.1016.j.cell.2012.01.035.

[155] Trends in Microbiology, Derrien M, Veigo P, Rethinking Diet to aid Human-Microbe Symbiosis, February 2017, vol 25, no 2, 100-112, doi:10.1016/j.tim.2016.09.011.

[156] Nutrients, Klimenko NS, Tyakht AV, Popenko AS, et al. Microbiome Responses to an Uncontrolled Short-Term Diet Intervention in the Frame of the Citizen Science Project, May 2018, vol 10, no 5, 576, doi:10.3390/nu10050576.

[157] Nutrients, Klimenko NS, Tyakht AV, Popenko AS, et al. Microbiome Responses to an Uncontrolled Short-Term Diet Intervention in the Frame of the Citizen Science Project, May 2018, vol 10, no 5, 576, doi:10.3390/nu10050576.

[158] Nutrients, Klimenko NS, Tyakht AV, Popenko AS, et al. Microbiome Responses to an Uncontrolled Short-Term Diet Intervention in the Frame of the Citizen Science ProjectMay 2018, vol 10, no 5, 576, doi:10.3390/nu10050576.

[159] Nutrients, Klimenko NS, Tyakht AV, Popenko AS, et al. Microbiome Responses to an Uncontrolled Short-Term Diet Intervention in the Frame of the Citizen Science ProjectMay 2018, vol 10, no 5, 576, doi:10.3390/nu10050576.

[160] Proceedings of the National Academy of Sciences of the United States of America, De Filippo C, Cavalieri D, Di Paola M, et al. Impact of Diet in Shaping gut Microbiota Revealed by a Comparative Study in Children from Europe and Rural Africa, August 17, 2010, vol 107, no 33, 14691-14696, doi:10.1073/pnas.1005963107.

[161] Philosophical Transactions of the Royal Society of London, Series B, Biological Sciences, Rolhion N, Chassaing B, When Pathogenic Bacteria Meet the Intestinal Microbiota, November 5, 2016, vol 37, no 1, 1707, doi:10.1098/rstb.2015.0504.

[162] European Heart Journal, Menni C, Lin C, Cecelia M, et al. Gut Microbial

Diversity is Associated with Lower Arterial Stiffness in Women, July 1, 2018, vo 39, no 25, 2390-2397, doi:10,1093/eurheartj/ehy226

[163] Gut, Manichanh C, Rigottier-Gois L, Bonnaud E, et al. Reduced Diversity of Faecal Microbiota in Crohn's Disease Revealed by a Metagenomic Approach, February 2006, vol 55, no 2, 205-211, doi:10.1136/gut.2005.073817.

[164] The Journal of Allergy and Clinical Immunology, Wang M, Karlsson C, Olsson C, et al. Reduced Diversity in the Early Fecal Microbiota of Infants with Atopic Eczema, January 2008, vol 121, no 1, 129-134, doi:10.1016/j.jaci.2007.09.011.

[165] Diabetes, de Goffau M, Luopajarvi K, Knip M, et al. Fecal Microbiota Composition Differs Between Children with B-Cell Autoimmunity and Those Without, April 2013, vol 62, no 4, 1238-1244, doi:10.2337/db12-0526.

[166] Journal of Diabetes and Obesity, Lambeth S, Carson T, Lowe J, et al. Composition, Diversity and Abundance of Gut Microbiome in Prediabetes and Type 2 Diabetes, December 26, 2015, vol 2, no 3, 1-7, doi:10.15436/2376-0949.15.031.

[167] Arthritis & Rheumatology, Scher J, Ubeda C, Artacho A, et al. Decreased Bacterial Diversity Characterizes an Altered Gut Microbiota in Psoriatic Arthritis and Resembles Dysbiosis of Inflammatory Bowel Disease, January 2015, vol 67, no 1, 128-139, doi:10.1002/art.38892.

[168] Nature, Turnbaugh PJ, Hamady M, Yatsunenko T, et al. A Core gut Microbiome in Obese and Lean Twins, January 22, 2009, vol 457, no 7228, 480-484, doi:10.1038/nature07540.

[168] Inflammation & Allergy - Drug Targets, Actis GC, The gut Microbiome, 2014, vol 13, no 4, 217-223, doi:10.2174/1871528113666140623113221.

[169] Inflammation & Allergy - Drug Targets, Actis GC, The gut Microbiome, 2014, vol 13, no 4, 217-223, doi:10.2174/1871528113666140623113221.

[170] Journal of Alternative and Complementary Medicine, Mc Dougall J, Bruce B, Spiller G, Westerdahl J, et al. Effects of a Very low-fat Diet in Subjects with Rheumatoid Arthritis, February 2002, vol 8, no 1, 71-75, doi:10.1089/107555302753507195.

[171] PLoS Medicine,Satija A, Bhupathiraju SN, Rimm EB, et al. Plant-Based Dietary Patterns and Incidence of Type 2 Diabetes in US Men and Women: Results From Three Prospective Cohort Studies, June 14, 2016, vol 13, no 6, doi:10.1371/journal.pmed.1002039. ecollection

[172] PLoS Medicine,Satija A, Bhupathiraju SN, Rimm EB, et al. Plant-Based Dietary Patterns and Incidence of Type 2 Diabetes in US Men and Women: Results From Three Prospective Cohort Studies, June 14, 2016, vol 13, no 6, doi:10.1371/journal.pmed.1002039. ecollection

[173] Cell Reports, Martinez I, Stegen JC, Maldonado-Gomez MX, et al. The gut Microbiota of Rural New Guineans: Composition, Diversity Patterns, and Ecological Processes, April 28, 2015, vol 11, no 4, 527-538, doi:10.1016/j.celrep.2015.03.049

[174] Cell Reports, Martinez I, Stegen JC, Maldonado-Gomez MX, et al. The gut Microbiota of Rural New Guineans: Composition, Diversity Patterns, and Ecological Processes, April 28, 2015, vol 11, no 4, 527-538, doi:10.1016/j.celrep.2015.03.049

[175] Science Advances, Clemente JC, Pehrsson EC, Blaser MJ, et al. The Microbiome of Uncontacted Ameridians, April 3, 2015, vol 1, no 3, pii: e1500183, doi:10. 1126/sciadv.1500183.

[176] Science Advances, Clemente JC, Pehrsson EC, Blaser MJ, et al. The Microbiome of Uncontacted Ameridians, April 3, 2015, vol 1, no 3, pii: e1500183, doi:10. 1126/sciadv.1500183.

The Gut Microbiota and Your Brain

[177] Molecular Endocrinology, Clarke G, Stilling RM, Kennedy PJ, et al. Minireview: Gut Microbiota: The Neglected Endocrine Organ, Aug 2014, vol 28, no 8, 1221-1238, doi:10.1210/me.2014-1108.

[178] The Proceeding of the Nutrition Society, Russell WR, Duncan SH, Flint HJ, The Gut Microbial Metabolome: Modulation of Cancer Risk in Obese Individuals, Feb 2013, vol 72, no 1, 178-188, doi:10.1017/S0029665112002881.

[179] Cell Host & Microbe, Wlodarska M, Luo C, Kolde R, et al. Indoleacrylic Acid Produced by Commensal Peptostreptococcus Species Suppresses Inflammation, July 12, 2017,vol 22, no 1, 25-37, doi:10.1016/j.chom.2017.06.007.

[180] Proceedings of the National Academy of Sciences of the United States of America, Wikoff WR, Anfora AT, Liu J, et al. Metabolomics Analysis Reveals Large Effects of Gut Microflora on Mammalian Blood Metabolites, March 10, 2009, vol 106, no 10, 3698-3703, doi:10.1073/pna.0812874106.

[181] Journal of Medicinal Food, Leo Galland, The Gut Microbiome and the Brain, December 1, 2014, vol 17, no 12, 1261-1272, doi:10.1089/jmf.2014.7000.

[182] Journal of Medicinal Food, Galland L, The Gut Microbiome and the Brain, Dec 1, 2014, 17(12), 1261-1272, doi:10.1089/jmf.2014.700.

[183] Journal of Medicinal Food, Galland L, The Gut Microbiome and the Brain, Dec 1, 2014, 17(12), 1261-1272, doi: 10.1089/jmf.2014.700

[184] Cellular and Molecular Life Sciences, Westfall S, Lomis N, Kahouli I, et al. Microbiome, Probiotics and Neurodegenerative Diseases: Deciphering the Gut Brain Axis, October 2017, vol 74, no 20, 3769-3787, doi:10.1007/s10018-017-2550-9.

[185] International Journal of Molecular Sciences, Caputi V, Giron MC, Microbiome-Gut-Brain Axis and Toll-Like Receptors in Parkinsos's Disease, June 6, 2018, vol 19, no 6, doi:10.3390/ijms19061689.

[186] Annals of the New York Academy f Sciences, Sherwin E, Dinan TG, Cryan JF, Recent Developments in Understanding the Role of the Gut Microbiome in Brain Health and Disease, May 2018, vol 1420, no 1, 5-25, doi:10.1111/nyas.13416.

[187] Scientific Reports, Vogt NM, Kerby RL, Dill-McFarland KA, et al. Gut Microbiome Alterations in Alzheimer's Disease, online Oct 19, 2017, doi:10.1038/s41598-017-13601-y.

[188] Scientific Reports, Vogt NM, Kerby RL, Dill-McFarland KA, et al. Gut Microbiome Alterations in Alzheimer's Disease, online Oct 19, 2017, doi:10.1038/s41598-017-13601-y.

[189] Scientific Reports, Vogt NM, Kerby RL, Dill-McFarland KA, et al. Gut Microbiome Alterations in Alzheimer's Disease, online Oct 19, 2017, doi:10.1038/s41598-017-13601-y.

[190] Alzheimer's & Dementia, the Journal of the Alzheimer's Association, MahmoudianDehkordi S, Arnold M, Nho K, et al. Altered Bile Acid Profile Associates with Cognitive Impairment in Alzheimer's Disease – An Emerging Role for Gut Microbiome, Jan 2019, vol 15, no 1, 76-92, doi:10.1016/j.jalz.2018.07.217.

[191] Movement Disorders: official journal of the Movement Disorder Society, Keshavarzian A, Green SJ, Engen PA, et al. Colonic Bacterial Composition in Parkinson's Disease, Sep 2015, vol 30, no 10, 1351-1360, doi:10.1002/mds.26307.

[192] Movement Disorders: official journal of the Movement Disorder Society, Keshavarzian A, Green SJ, Engen PA, et al. Colonic Bacterial Composition in Parkinson's Disease, Sep 2015, vol 30, no 10, 1351-1360,

doi:10.1002/mds.26307.

[193] Movement Disorders: official journal of the Movement Disorder Society, Keshavarzian A, Green SJ, Engen PA, et al. Colonic Bacterial Composition in Parkinson's Disease, Sep 2015, vol 30, no 10, 1351-1360, doi:10.1002/mds.26307.

[194] PLoS One, Larsen N Vogensen FK, van den Berg FW, et al. Gut Microbiota in Human Adults With Type 2 Diabetes Differs From Non-Diabetic Adults, Feb 5, 2010, vol 5, no 2, e9085, doi:10.1371/journal.pone.0009085.

[195] The European Journal of Neuroscience, Lebouvier T, Chaumette T, Paillusson S, et al. The Second Brain and Parkinson's Disease, Sep 2009, vol 30, no 5, 735-741, doi:10.1111/j.1460-9568.2009.06873.x.

[196] World Journal of Gastroenterology, Awad RA, Neurogenic Bowel Dysfunction in Patients with Spinal Cord Injury, Myelomeningocele, Multiple Sclerosis and Parkinson's, Dec 14, 2011, vol 17, no 46, 5035-5048, doi:10.3748/wjg.v17.j46.5035.

[197] PLoS One, Forsyth CB, Shannon KM, Kordower JH, et al. Increased Intestinal Permeability Correlates with Sigmoid Mucosa Alpha-Synuclein Staining and Endotoxin Exposure Markers in Early Parkinson's Disease, 2011, vol 6, no 12, e28032, doi:10.1371/journal.pone.0028032.

[198] PLoS One, Forsyth CB, Shannon KM, Kordower JH, et al. Increased Intestinal Permeability Correlates with Sigmoid Mucosa Alpha-Synuclein Staining and Endotoxin Exposure Markers in Early Parkinson's Disease, 2011, vol 6, no 12, e28032, doi:10.1371/journal.pone.0028032.

[199] Biological Psychiatry, Swardfager W, Lanctot K, Rothenburg L, et al. A Meta-Analysis of Cytokines in Alzheimer's Disease, November 15, 2010, vol68, no10, doi:10.1016/j.biopsych.2010.06.012

[200] JAMA Neurology, Qin XY, Zhang SP, Cao C, et al. Aberrations in Peripheral Inflammatory Cytokine Levels in Parkinson's Disease: A Systematic Review and Meta-Analysis, November 1 2016, vol 73, no 11, 1316-1324, doi:10.1001/jamaneurol.2016.2742.

[201] Journal of Diabetes Science and Technology, de la Monte SM, Wands JR, Alzheimer's Disease is Type 3 Diabetes- Evidence Reviewed, Nov 2008, vol 2 no 6, 1101-1113, doi:10.1177/193229680800200619.

[202] Journal of Diabetes Science and Technology, de la Monte SM, Wands JR, Alzheiler's Disease is Type 3 Diabetes- Evidence Reviewed, Nov 2008, vol 2 no 6, 1101-1113, doi:10.1177/193229680800200619.

Your Microbiome Affects Your Liver and Your Liver Affects Your Microbiome

[203] Biochemistry Research International, Degli Esposti D, Hamelin J, Bosselut N, et al. Mitochndrial Roles and Cytoprotection in Chronic Liver Injury, April 11, 2012, vol 2012, 387626, doi:10.1155/2012/387626.

[204] Current Neuropharmacology, Shukla M, Govitrapong P, Boontem P, et al. Mechanisms of Melatonin in Alleviating Alzheimer's Disease, October 2017, vol 15, no 7, 1010-1031, doi:10.2174/1570159x15666170313123454.

[205] Pharmacological Research, Vincent B, Protective Roles of Melatonin Agaianst the Amyloid-Dependent Developmentof Alzheimer's Disease: A Critical Review, August 2018, vol 134, 223-237, doi:10.1016/j.phrs.2018.06.011.

[206] Journal of Pineal Research, Shukla M, Htoo HH, Wintachai P, et al. Melatonin Stimulates the Nonamyloidogenic Processin of BAPP Through the Positive Transcriptional Regulation of ADAM10 andADAM17, March 2015, vol 58, no 2, 151-165, doi:10.1111/jpi.12200.

[207] Free Radical Biology and Medicine, Yan MH, Wang X, Zhu X, Mitochondrial Defects and Oxidative Stress in Alzheimer's Disease and Parkinson's Disease, September 2013, vol 62, 90-101, doi:10.1016/j.freeradbiomed.2012.11.014.

[208] Frontiers in Bioscience, Onyango IG, Khan SM, Bennett JP Jr, Mitochondria in the Pathophysiology of Alzheimer's and Parkinson's Diseases, Landmark Edition, January 1, 2017, vol 22, 854-872, doi:10.2741/4521.

[209] Free Radical Biology and Medicine, Yan MH, Wang X, Zhu X, Mitochondrial Defects and Oxidative Stress in Alzheimer's Disease and Parkinson's Disease, September 2013, vol 62, 90-101, doi:10.1016/j.freeradbiomed.2012.11.014.

[210] Frontiers in Bioscience, Onyango IG, Khan SM, Bennett JP Jr, Mitochondria in the Pathophysiology of Alzheimer's and Parkinson's Diseases, Landmark Edition, January 1, 2017, vol 22, 854-872, doi:10.2741/4521.

[211] Journal of Experimental Medicine, Gustafson BE, Lanke LS, Bilirubin and Urobilins in Germfree, Ex-Germfree, and Conventional Rats, November 30, 1960, vol 112, no 6, 076-981, doi:10.1084/jem.112.6.976.

[212] The Journal of Biological Chemistry, Gustafsson BE, Einarsson K, Gustafsson J, Influence of Cholesterol Feeding on Liver Micrcosomal Metabolism of Steroids and Bile Acids in Conventional and Germ-free rats, November 10, 1975, vol 250, no 21, 8496-8502, PMD:811655.

[213] Journal of Lipid Research, Kellogg TF, Wostmann BS, Fecal Neutral Steroids and Bile Acids From Germfree Rats, September 1969, vol10, no 5, 495-503, PMID:5808824.

[214] Nature Medicine, Seki E, De Minicis S, Osterreicher Ch, et al. TLR4 Enhances TGF-beta Signaling and Hepatic Fibrosis, Nov 2007, 13(11):1324-1332, doi 10.1038/nm1663.

[215] British Journal of Pharmacology, Thiermermann C, Ruetten H, Wu CC, et al. The Multiple Organ Dysfunction Syndrome Caused by Endotoxin in the rat: Attenuation of Liver Dysfunction by Inhibitors of Nitric Oxide Synthase, Dec 1995, 116(7):2845-2851, doi:10.1111/j.1476-5381.1995,tb15935.x.

[216] British Journal of Pharmacology, Thiermermann C, Ruetten H, Wu CC, et al. The Multiple Organ Dysfunction Syndrome Caused by Endotoxin in the rat: Attenuation of Liver Dysfunction by Inhibitors of Nitric Oxide Synthase, Dec 1995, 116(7):2845-2851, doi:10.1111/j.1476-5381.1995,tb15935.x.

[217] Expert Review of Gastroenterology & Hepatology, Preveden T. Scarpellini E, Milic N, et al. Gut Microbiota Changes and Chronic Hepatitis C Virus Infection, September 2017, vol 11, no 9, 813-819, doi:10.1080/17474124.2017.1343663.

[218] Proceedings of the National Academy of Sciences of the United States of America, Dumas ME, Barton RH, Toye A, Metabolic Profiling Reveals a Contribution of Gut Microbiota to Fatty Liver Phenotype in Insulin-Resistant Mice, August 15, 2006, vol 103, no 33, 12511-12516, doi:10.1073/pnas.0601056103.

[219] Proceedings of the National Academy of Sciences of the United States of America, Dumas ME, Barton RH, Toye A, Metabolic Profiling Reveals a Contribution of Gut Microbiota to Fatty Liver Phenotype in Insulin-Resistant Mice, August 15, 2006, vol 103, no 33, 12511-12516, doi:10.1073/pnas.0601056103.

[220] Journal of Gastroenterology and Hepatology, Sato N, Central Role of Mitchondria in Metabolic Regulation of Liver Pathophysiology, June 2007, vol 22, suppl 1, S1-6, doi:10.1111/j.1440-1746.2007.04963.x.

[221] Gastroenterology, Charlton MR, Burns JM, Pedersen RA, et al. Frequency and Outcomes of Liver Transplantation for Nonalcoholic Steatohepatitis in the United States, Oct 2011, vol 141 no 4, 1249-1253, doi:10.1053/j.hastro.2011.06.061.

[222] Journal of Digestive Diseases, Mc Cullough AJ, Epidemiology of the Metabolic Syndrome in the USA, Oct 2011, vol 12, no 5, 333-340, doi:10.1111/j.1751-2980.2010.00469.x.
[223] Plos One, Lytle KA, Jump DB, Is Western Diet-Induced Nonalcoholic Steatohepatitis in Ldlr-/- Mice Reversible?, Jan 13, 2016, https://doi.org/10.1371/journal.pone.0146942.

Vital Factors for Your Health

[224] The Journal of the American Medical Association, Welsh J A, Sharma A, Abramson J L, et al. Caloric Sweetener Consumption and Dyslipidemia Among US Adults, April 21, 2010;303(15):1490-1497, doi:10.1001/jama.2010.449.
[225] The Journal of the American Medical Association, Welsh J A, Sharma A, Abramson J L, et al. Caloric Sweetener Consumption and Dyslipidemia Among US Adults, April 21, 2010;303(15):1490-1497, doi:10.1001/jama.2010.449.
[226] Center for Disease Control, National Center for Health Statistics, National Health and Nutrition Examination Survey 2011-2012, 2013-2014, Rosinger A Phd, MPH, Herrick K PhD, MSc, Gahche J MPH, et al. Sugar Sweetened Beverage Consumption Among US Adults, 2011-2014, NCHS Data Brief No. 270, January 2017, https://www.cdc.gov/nchs/products/databriefs/db270.htm.
[227] United States Department of Agriculture, Agriculture Research Service, Raatz Susan, The Question of Sugar, News 2012, https://www.ars.usda.gov/plains-area/gfnd/gfhnrc/docs/news-2012/the-question-of-sugar/.
[228] United States Department of Agriculture, Table 19-US. cane and beet sugar deliveries, monthly, quarterly and by fiscal and calendar year, Oct 1991-3/29/2019.
[229] United States Department of Agriculture, Table 19-US. cane and beet sugar deliveries, monthly, quarterly and by fiscal and calendar year, Oct 1991-3/29/2019.
[230] United States Department of Agriculture, Table 19-US. cane and beet sugar deliveries, monthly, quarterly and by fiscal and calendar year, Oct 1991-3/29/2019.
[231] United States Department of Agriculture, Table 19-US. cane and beet sugar deliveries, monthly, quarterly and by fiscal and calendar year, Oct 1991-3/29/2019.
[232] United States Department of Agriculture, Table 19-US. cane and beet sugar deliveries, monthly, quarterly and by fiscal and calendar year, Oct 1991-3/29/2019.
[233] United States Department of Agriculture, Table 19-US. cane and beet sugar deliveries, monthly, quarterly and by fiscal and calendar year, Oct 1991-3/29/2019.
[234] United States Department of Agriculture, Table 19-US. cane and beet sugar deliveries, monthly, quarterly and by fiscal and calendar year, Oct 1991-3/29/2019.
[235] United States Department of Agriculture, Table 19-US. cane and beet sugar deliveries, monthly, quarterly and by fiscal and calendar year, Oct 1991-3/29/2019.
[236] United States Department of Agriculture, Table 19-US. cane and beet sugar deliveries, monthly, quarterly and by fiscal and calendar year, Oct 1991-3/29/2019.
[237] United States Department of Agriculture, Table 19-US. cane and beet sugar deliveries, monthly, quarterly and by fiscal and calendar year, Oct 1991-

3/29/2019.
[238] United States Department of Agriculture, Table 19-US. cane and beet sugar deliveries, monthly, quarterly and by fiscal and calendar year, Oct 1991-3/29/2019.
[239] United States Department of Agriculture, Table 19-US. cane and beet sugar deliveries, monthly, quarterly and by fiscal and calendar year, Oct 1991-3/29/2019.
[240] Center for Disease Control, National Center for Health Statistics, National Health and Nutrition Examination Survey 2011-2012, 2013-2014, Rosinger A Phd, MPH, Herrick K PhD, MSc, Gahche J MPH, et al. Sugar Sweetened Beverage Consumption Among US Adults, 2011-2014, NCHS Data Brief No. 270, January 2017, https://www.cdc.gov/nchs/products/databriefs/db270.htm.
[241] Boston Public Health Commission, Health Effects of Sugary Drinks, http://www.bphc.org/whatwedo/healthy-eating-active-living/sugar-smarts/be-sugar-smart/Pages/Health-Effects-of-Sugary-Drinks.aspx.
[242] Circulation, American Heart Association, Malik V ScD, Li Y PhD, Pan A PhD, et al. Long-Term Consumption of Sugar- Sweetened Beverages and Artificially Sweetened Beverages and Risk of Mortality in US Adults,. April 30, 2019, 2019;139:2113–2125,   doi: 10.1161/CIRCULATIONAHA.118.037401.
[243] Circulation, American Heart Association, Malik V ScD, Li Y PhD, Pan A PhD, et al. Long-Term Consumption of Sugar- Sweetened Beverages and Artificially Sweetened Beverages and Risk of Mortality in US Adults,. April 30, 2019, 2019;139:2113–2125. doi: 10.1161/CIRCULATIONAHA.118.037401.
[244]Circulation, American Heart Association, Malik V ScD, Li Y PhD, Pan A PhD, et al. Long-Term Consumption of Sugar- Sweetened Beverages and Artificially Sweetened Beverages and Risk of Mortality in US Adults,. April 30, 2019, 2019;139:2113–2125. doi: 10.1161/CIRCULATIONAHA.118.037401.
[245] Circulation, American Heart Association, Malik V ScD, Li Y PhD, Pan A PhD, et al. Long-Term Consumption of Sugar- Sweetened Beverages and Artificially Sweetened Beverages and Risk of Mortality in US Adults,. April 30, 2019, 2019;139:2113–2125. doi: 10.1161/CIRCULATIONAHA.118.037401.
[246] Center for Disease Control, National Center for Health Statistics, National Health and Nutrition Examination Survey 2011-2012, 2013-2014, Rosinger A Phd, MPH, Herrick K PhD, MSc, Gahche J MPH, et al. Sugar Sweetened Beverage Consumption Among US Adults, 2011-2014, NCHS Data Brief No. 270, January 2017, https://www.cdc.gov/nchs/products/databriefs/db270.htm.
[247] Center for Disease Control, National Center for Health Statistics, National Health and Nutrition Examination Survey 2011-2012, 2013-2014, Rosinger A Phd, MPH, Herrick K PhD, MSc, Gahche J MPH, et al. Sugar Sweetened Beverage Consumption Among US Adults, 2011-2014, NCHS Data Brief No. 270, January 2017, https://www.cdc.gov/nchs/products/databriefs/db270.htm.
[248] Center for Disease Control, National Center for Health Statistics, National Health and Nutrition Examination Survey 2011-2012, 2013-2014, Rosinger A Phd, MPH, Herrick K PhD, MSc, Gahche J MPH, et al. Sugar Sweetened Beverage Consumption Among US Adults, 2011-2014, NCHS Data Brief No. 270, January 2017, https://www.cdc.gov/nchs/products/databriefs/db270.htm.
[249] Center for Disease Control, National Center for Health Statistics, National Health and Nutrition Examination Survey 2011-2012, 2013-2014, Rosinger A Phd, MPH, Herrick K PhD, MSc, Gahche J MPH, et al. Sugar Sweetened Beverage Consumption Among US Adults, 2011-2014, NCHS Data Brief No. 270, January 2017, https://www.cdc.gov/nchs/products/databriefs/db270.htm.
[250] The American Journal of Clinical Nutrition, Duffey K, Gordon-Larsen P, Steffen L, et al. Drinking Caloric Beverages Increases the Risk of Adverse

Cardiometabolic Outcomes in the Coronary Artery Risk Development in Young Adults (CARDIA) Study, Oct 1 2010, 92 (4), 954-959, doi.org/10.3945/ajcn.2010.29478.

[251] CARDIA, https://www.cardia.dopm.uab.edu/.

[252] The Journal of the American Medical Association, Welsh J A, Sharma A, Abramson J L, et al. Caloric Sweetener Consumption and Dyslipidemia Among US Adults, April 21, 2010;303(15):1490-1497, doi:10.100/jama.2010.449

[253] The Journal of the American Medical Association , Kearns CE, Schmidt LA, Glantz SA, Sugar Industry and Coronary Heart Disease Research A Historical Analysis of Internal Industry Documents, Nov 1 , 2016, 176(11): 1680-1685, doi:10.1001/jamainternmed.2016.5394.

[254] The Journal of the American Medical Association , Kearns CE, Schmidt LA, Glantz SA, Sugar Industry and Coronary Heart Disease Research A Historical Analysis of Internal Industry Documents, Nov 1 , 2016, 176(11): 1680-1685, doi:10.1001/jamainternmed.2016.5394.

[255] The Journal of the American Medical Association , Kearns CE, Schmidt LA, Glantz SA, Sugar Industry and Coronary Heart Disease Research A Historical Analysis of Internal Industry Documents, Nov 1 , 2016, 176(11): 1680-1685, doi:10.1001/jamainternmed.2016.5394.

[256] The Journal of the American Medical Association , Kearns CE, Schmidt LA, Glantz SA, Sugar Industry and Coronary Heart Disease Research A Historical Analysis of Internal Industry Documents, Nov 1 , 2016, 176(11): 1680-1685, doi:10.1001/jamainternmed.2016.5394.

[257] PLoS Biology (Public Library of Science), Kearns CE, Apollonio D, Glantz SA, The Sugar Industry Sponsorship of Germ-Free Rodent Studies Linking Sucrose to Hyperlipidemia and Cancer: A Historical Analysis of Internal Documents, Nov 2017, 15(11): e2003460, doi:10.1371/journal.pbio.2003460.

[258] PLoS Biology (Public Library of Science), Kearns CE, Apollonio D, Glantz SA, The Sugar Industry Sponsorship of Germ-Free Rodent Studies Linking Sucrose to Hyperlipidemia and Cancer: A Historical Analysis of Internal Documents, Nov 2017, 15(11): e2003460, doi:10.1371/journal.pbio.2003460.

[259] PLoS Biology (Public Library of Science), Kearns CE, Apollonio D, Glantz SA, The Sugar Industry Sponsorship of Germ-Free Rodent Studies Linking Sucrose to Hyperlipidemia and Cancer: A Historical Analysis of Internal Documents, Nov 2017, 15(11): e2003460, doi:10.1371/journal.pbio.2003460.

[260] Applied Microbiology and Biotechnology, Yu X, Wu X, Qiu L, et al. Analysis of the Intestinal Microbial Community Structure of Healthy and Long-living Elderly Residents in Gaotian Village of Liuyang City, November 2015, vol 99, no 21, 9085-9095, doi:10.1007/s00253-015-6888-3.

Vary Your Foods

[261] Nutrients, Conlon MA, Bird AR, The Impact of Diet and Lifestyle on the gut Microbiota and Human Health, January 2015, vol 7, no 1, 17-44, doi:10.3390/nu7010017.

[262] Proceedings of the National Academy of Sciences of the United States of America, Frank DN, St Amand AL, Feldman RA, et al. Molecular- Phylogenetic Characterization of Microbial Community Imbalances in Human Inflammatory Bowel Diseases, August 21, 2007, vol 104, no 34, 13780-13785, doi:10.1073/pnas.0706625104.

[263] The Journal of Allergy and Clinical Immunology, Gore C, Munro K, Lay C, et al. Bifidobacterium Pseudocatenulatum is Associated with Atopic Eczema: a

Nested Case-Control Study Investigating the Fecal Microbiota of Infants, January 2008, vol 121, no 1, 136-140. Doi:101016/j.jaci.2007.07.061.
[264] Environmental Microbiology Reports, Nava GM, Carbonero F, Ou J, et al. Hydrogenotrophic Microbiota Distinguish Native Africans From African and European Americans, June 2012, vol 4, no 3, 307-315, doi:10.1111/j.1758-2229.2012.0034.x.
[265] Environmental Microbiology Reports, Nava GM, Carbonero F, Ou J, et al. Hydrogenotrophic Microbiota Distinguish Native Africans From African and European Americans, June 2012, vol 4, no 3, 307-315, doi:10.1111/j.1758-2229.2012.0034.x.
[266] Environmental Microbiology Reports, Nava GM, Carbonero F, Ou J, et al. Hydrogenotrophic Microbiota Distinguish Native Africans From African and European Americans, June 2012, vol 4, no 3, 307-315, doi:10.1111/j.1758-2229.2012.0034.x.
[267] Nutrients, Conlon M A, Bird A R, The Impact of Diet and Lifestyle on Gut Microbiota and Human Health, January 2015, vol 7, no 1, 17-44, doi:10.13390/nu7010017
[268] Environmental Microbiology Reports, Nava GM, Carbonero F, Ou J, et al. Hydrogenotrophic Microbiota Distinguish Native Africans From African and European Americans, June 2012, vol 4, no 3, 307-315, doi:10.1111/j.1758-2229.2012.0034.x.

Phytonutrients - What Are They?

[269] Proceedings of the National Academy of Sciences of the United States of America, Bansal T, Alaniz RC, Wood TK, et al. The Bacterial Signal Indole Increases Epithelial-Cell Tight-Junction Resistance and Attenuates Indicators of Inflammation, January 5, 2010, vol 107, no 1, 228-233, doi:10.1073/pnas.0906112107
[270] Applied and Environmental Microbiology, Sabag-Daigle A, Soares JA, Smith JN, et al. The Acyl Homoserine Lactone Receptor, SdiA, of Escherichia coli and Salmonella Enterica Serovar Typhimurium Does not Respond to Indole, August 2012, vol 78, no 15, 5424-5431, doi:10.1128/AEM.00046-12.
[271] The Journal of Gene Medicine, Kanerva A, Raki M, Ranki T et al. Chlorpromazine and Apigenin Reduce Adenovirus Replication and Decrease Replication Associated Toxicity, January 2007, vol 9 no 1, 3-9, doi:10.1002/jgm.984.
[272] Natural Product Research, Zhou L, Li D, Wang J, et al. Antibacterial Phenolic Compounds From the Spines of Gleditsia Sinensis Lam, May 2007, vol 21, no 4, 283-291, doi: 10.1080/14786410701192637.
[273] Molecular Nutrition & Food Research, Friedman M, Overview of Antibacterial, Antitoxin, Antiviral, and Antifungal Activities of Tea Flavonoids and Teas, January 2007, vol 51, no 1, 116-134, doi: 10.1002/mnfr2006.200600173.
[274] European Journal of Medical Chemistry, Nowakowska Z, A Review of Anti-Infective and Anti-Inflammatory Chalcones, February 2007, vol 42, no 2, 125-137, doi: 10.1016.ejmech.2006.09.019.
[275]Cancer Detection and Prevention, Hostanska K, Jurgenliemk G, Abel G, et al. Willow Bark Extract (BNO1455) and its Fractions Suppress Growth and Induce Apoptosis in Human Colon and Lung Cancer Cells, April 2007, vol 31 no 2, 129-39, doi:10.1016/j.cdp.2007.03.001.
[276] Clinical Pharmacology and Therapeutics, Wagner I, Greim C, Laufer S, et al. Influence of Willow Bark Extract on Cyclooxygenase Acitivity and on Tumor Necrosis Factor Alpha or Interleukin 1 Beta Release in Vitro and Ex Vivo, March

2003, vol 73, no 3, 272-274, doi: 10.1067/mcp.2003.32.
[277] American Journal of Cancer Research, Aghajanpour M, Reza Nazer M Obeidavi Z, et al. Functional Foods and Their Role in Cancer Prevention and Health Promotion: a Comprehensive Review, April 1, 2017, vol 7, no 4, 740-769. PMCID PMC5411786.
[278] Nutrients, Selvakumar P, Badgeley A, Murphy P, et al. Flavonoids and Polyphenols Act as Epigenetic Modifiers in Breast Cancer, Mar 13, 2020, vol 12, no 3, pii:E761, doi:10.3390/nu12030761.
[279] Circulation, Ma L, Liu G, Ding M, et al. Isoflavone Intake and the Risk of Coronary Heart Disease in US Men and Women: Results From 3 Prospective Cohort Studies, Apr 7, 2020, vol 141, no 14, 1127-1137, doi:10.1161/CIRCULATIONAHA.119.041306.
[280] Pharmacognosy Review, Kalaiselvan V, Kalaivani M, Vijayakumar A, et al. Current Knowledge and Future Direction of Research on Soy Isoflavones as a Therapeutic Agents, Jul-Dec 2010, vol 4, no 8, 111-117, doi:10.4103/0973-7847.70900.
[281] Watson Ronald Ross, Preedy Victor R, eds. Fruits, Vegetables, and Herbs. Academic Press, Elsevier, 2016, doi.org/10.1016/C2015-0-01705-1.
[282] Pharmacognosy Review, Kalaiselvan V, Kalaivani M, Vijayakumar A, et al. Current Knowledge and Future Direction of Research on Soy Isoflavones as a Therapeutic Agents, Jul-Dec 2010, vol 4, no 8, 111-117, doi:10.4103/0973-7847.70900.
[283] Gwaltney-Brant Sharon M, contributor in Nutraceuticals: Efficacy, Safety, ad Toxicity. Academic Press, Elsevier, 2016, 87-99, doi.org/10.1016/B978-0-12-802147-7.00007-3.
[284] Gwaltney-Brant Sharon M, contributor in Nutraceuticals: Efficacy, Safety, ad Toxicity. Academic Press, Elsevier, 2016, 87-99, doi.org/10.1016/B978-0-12-802147-7.00007-3.
[285] Current Cardiology Reviews, Sekikawa A, Ihara M, Lopez O, et al. Effect of S-equol and Soy Isoflavones on Heart and Brain, 2019, vol 15, no 2, 114-135, doi:10.2174/1573403X15666181205104717.
[286] International Journal of Molecular Sciences, Seo JY, Kim BR, Oh J, et al.Soybean-Derived Phytoalexins Improve Cognitive Function Through Activation of Nrf2/HO-1 Signaling Pathway, Jan 2018, vol 19, no 1, 268, doi:10.3390/ijms19010268.
[287] Cytokine, Mirahmadi SM, Shahmohammadi A, Rousta AM, et al. Soy Isoflavone Genistein Attenuates Lipopolysaccharide-Induced Cognitive Impairments in the ratvia Exerting Anti-Oxidative and Anti-Inflammatory Effects, Apr 2018, vol 104, 151-159, doi:10.1016/j.cyto.2017.10.008.
[288] International Journal of Molecular Sciences, de Camargo AC, Favero BT, Morzelle MC, et al. Is Chcikpea a Potential Substitute for Soybean?, Phenolic Bioactives and Potential Health Benefits, May 29, vol 20, no 11, doi:10.3390/ijms20112644 2019.
[289] Experimental Physiology, Ballman C, Denney T, Beyers RJ, et al. Long-term Dietary Quercetin Enrichment as a Cardioprotective Countermeasure in MDX Mice, June 1 2017, vol 102 no 6, 635-649, doi:10.1113/EP086091.
[290] European Journal of Medicinal Chemistry, Patel RV, Mistry BM, Shinde SK, et al. Therapeutic Potential of Quercetin as a Cardiovascular Agent, July, 2018, vol 15, no 155, 889-904, doi:10.1016/j.ejmech.2018.06.053.
[291] Toxicology and Applied Pharmacology, Veith C, Drent M, Bast A, et al. The Disturbed Redox Balance in Pulmonary Fibrosis is Modulated by the Plant Falvonoid Quercetin, December 1,2017, no 336, 40-48, doi:10.1016/j.taap.2017.10.001.
[292] Advances in Neurobiology, Elumalai P, Lakshim S, Role of Quercetin Benefits

in Neurodegeneration, 2016, no12, 229-245, doi:10.1007/978-3-319-28383-8_12.

[293] Journal of Neurochemistry, Av M, Luo J, Lnaglev M, et al. Molecular Mechanisms Underlying Protective Effects of Quercetin Against Mitochondrial Dysfunction and ProgressiveDopamminergic Neurodegeneration in Cell Culture and MitoPark Transgenic Mouse Models of Parkinson's Disease, June 2017, vol 141, no 5, 766-782, doi:10.1111.jnc:14033.

[294] Neurobiology of Aging, Baral S, Pariyar R, Kim J, et al. Quercetin-3-0-Glucuronide Promotes the Proliferation and Migration of Neural Stem Cells, April 2017, no 52, 39-52, doi:10.1016/j.neurobiolaging.2016.12.24.

[295] Oxidative Medicine and Cellular Longevity, Zhao Y, Chen B, Shen J, et al. The Beneficial Effects of Quercetin, Curcuma, and Resveratrol in Obesity, 2017, 1459497, doi:10.1155/2017/1459497.

[296] Nutrition Research (New York, N.Y.), Carvalho FB, Gutierres JM, Beckman D, et al. Quercetin Treatment Regulates the Na+, K+ -ATPase Acitivity, Peripheral Cholinergic Enzymes, and Oxidative Stress in a Rat Model of Demylenation, July 2018, no 55, 45-56, doi:10.1016/nutres.2018.04.004.

[297] Toxicology and Applied Pharmacology, Veith C, Drent M, Bast A, et al. The Disturbed Redox Balance in Pulmonary Fibrosis is Modulated by the Plant Falvonoid Quercetin, December 1,2017, no 336, 40-48, doi:10.1016/j.taap.2017.10.001.

[298] Mini Reviews in Medicinal Chemistry, Bai X, Yao L, Ma X, et al. Small Molecules as SIRT Modulators,2018, vol 18 no 13, 1151-1157, doi:10.2174/1389557516666160620095103.

[299] Molecules, Marunaka Y, Marunaka R, Sun H, et al. Actions of Quercetin, a Polyphenol, on Blood Pressure, January 2017, vol22, no 2, pii:E209, doi:10.3390/molecules22020209.

[300] Pharmacological Research, Perez A, Gonzalez-Manzano S, Jimenez R, et al. The Flavonoid Quercetin Induces Acute Vasodilator Effects in Healthy Volunteers: Correlation with Beta-Glucuronidase Activity, November 2014, no 89, 11-18, doi:10.1016/j.phrs.2014.07.005

[301] Molecular Nutrition & Food Research, Bondonno NP, Bondonno CP, Blekkenhorst LC, et al. Flavonoid-Ric Apple Improves Endothelial Function in Individuals at Risk for Cardiovascular Disease: A Randomized Controlled Clinical Trial, February 2018, vol 62, no 3, doi:10.1002/mnh.201700674.

[302] Molecular Nutrition & Food Research, Bondonno NP, Bondonno CP, Blekkenhorst LC, et al. Flavonoid-Ric Apple Improves Endothelial Function in Individuals at Risk for Cardiovascular Disease: A Randomized Controlled Clinical Trial, February 2018, vol 62, no 3, doi:10.1002/mnh.201700674.

[303] European Journal of Medicinal Chemistry, Patel RV, Mistry BM, Shinde SK, et al. Therapeutic Potential of Quercetin as a Cardiovascular Agent, July, 2018, vol 15, no 155, 889-904, doi:10.1016/j.ejmech.2018.06.053.

[304] Current Topics in Medicinal Chemistry, Gormaz JG, Quentremil S, Rodrigo R, Cardiovascular Disease: A Target for the Pharmacological Effects of Quercetin, 2015, vol 15, no 17, 1735-1742, PMID25915608.

[305] British Journal of Cancer, Jones DJ, Lamb JH, Verschovie RD, et al. Characterisation of Metabolites of the Putative Cancer Chemopreventive Agent Quercetin and their Effect on Cyclo-Oxygenase Activity, September 13,2014, vol 91, no 6, 1213-1219, doi:10.1038/sj,bjc.6602091.

[306] Current Medicinal Chemistry, Brito AF, Ribeiro M, Abrantes AM, et al. Quercetin in Cancer Treatment, Alone or in Combination with Conventional Therapeutics?, 2015, vol 22 no 26, 3025-3039, PMID:2624923.

[307] Journal of Gastrointestinal Cancer, Haghi A, Azimi H, Rahimi R, A Comprehensive Review on Pharmacotheapeutics of Three Phytochemicals,

Curcumin, Quercetin, and Allicin, in the Treatment of Gastric Cancer, December 2017, vol 48, no 4, 314-320, doi:10.1007/s12029-017-9997-7.

[308] The Journal of Nutrition, Labbe D, Provencal M, Lamy S, et al. The Flavinoids Quercitin, Kaempferol, and Myricetin Inhibit Hepatocyte Growth Factor-Induced Medulloblastoma Cell Migration, April 2009, vol 139, no 4, 646-652, doi:10.3945/jn.108.102616.

[309] The Journal of Nutrition, Labbe D, Provencal M, Lamy S, et al. The Flavinoids Quercetin, Kaempferol, and Myricetin Inhibit Hepatocyte Growth Factor-Induced Medulloblastoma Cell Migration, April 2009, vol 139, no 4, 646-652, doi:10.3945/jn.108.102616.

[310] The Journal of Nutrition, Labbe D, Provencal M, Lamy S, et al. The Flavinoids Quercetin, Kaempferol, and Myricetin Inhibit Hepatocyte Growth Factor-Induced Medulloblastoma Cell Migration, April 2009, vol 139, no 4, 646-652, doi:10.3945/jn.108.102616.

[311] World Cancer Research Fund/American Institute for Cancer Research. Continuous Update Project Expert Report 2018. Wholegrains, Vegetables and Fruit and the Risk of Cancer. dietandcancerreprt.org

[312] World Cancer Research Fund/American Institute for Cancer Research. Continuous Update Project Expert Report 2018. Wholegrains, Vegetables and Fruit and the Risk of Cancer. dietandcancerreprt.org

The Rainbow of Phytonutrients

[313] Annual Review of Food Science and Technology, He J, Guisti MM, Anthocyanins: Natural Colorants with Health Promoting Properties, 2010, 1, 163-187. doi:10.1146/annurev.food.080708.100754.

[314] Annual Review of Food Science and Technology, He J, Guisti MM, Anthocyanins: Natural Colorants with Health Promoting Properties, 2010, 1, 163-187. doi:10.1146/annurev.food.080708.100754.

[315] Journal of Agricultural and Food Chemistry, Passamonti S, Vrhovsek U, Vanzo A, et al. Fast Access of Some Grape Pigments to the Brain, September 7, 2005, vol 53, no 18, 7029-7034, doi:10.1021/jf050565k.

[316] Journal of Agricultural and Food Chemistry ,Milbury PE, Kalt W, Xenobiotic Metabolism and Berry Flavonoids Transport Across the Blood-Brain Barrier, April 14, 2010, vol 58, no 7, 3950-3960, doi:10.1021/jf903529m.

[317] Journal of Agricultural and Food Chemistry, Kalt W, Blumberg JB, McDonald JE, et al. Identification of Anthocyanins in the Liver, Eye, and Brain of Blueberry-fed Pigs, February 13, 2008, vol 56, no 3, 705-712, doi:10.1021/jf071998l.

[318] Journal of Agricultural and Food Chemistry ,Milbury PE, Kalt W, Xenobiotic Metabolism and Berry Flavonoids Transport Across the Blood-Brain Barrier, April 14, 2010, vol 58, no 7, 3950-3960, doi:10.1021/jf903529m.

[319] Stroke, Oude Griep Linda M, Verschuren WM Monique, Kromhout Dann, et al., Colors of Fruits and Vegetables and 10-Year Incidence of Stroke, 2011, 42, 3190-3195. doi.org/10.1161/STROKEAHA.110.611152.

[320] Stroke, Oude Griep Linda M, Verschuren WM Monique, Kromhout Dann, et al., Colors of Fruits and Vegetables and 10-Year Incidence of Stroke, 2011, 42, 3190-3195. doi.org/10.1161/STROKEAHA.110.611152.

[321] Cancer, Ho WJ, Simon MS., Yildiz VO, et al. Antioxidant Micronutrients and the Risk of Renal Cell Carcinoma in the Women's Health Initiative Cohort, February 15, 2015, vol 121, issue 4, 580-588, doi:10.1002/cncr.29091.

[322] Annual Review of Food Science and Technology, He J, Guisti MM, Anthocyanins: Natural Colorants with Health Promoting Properties, 2010, 1,

163-187. doi:10.1146/annurev.food.080708.100754.

[323] Annual Review of Food Science and Technology, He J, Guisti MM, Anthocyanins: Natural Colorants with Health Promoting Properties, 2010, 1, 163-187. doi:10.1146/annurev.food.080708.100754.

[324] Journal of Agricultural and Food Chemistry, Passamonti S, Vrhovsek U, Vanzo A, et al. Fast Access of Some Grape Pigments to the Brain, September 7, 2005, vol 53, no 18, 7029-7034, doi:10.1021/jf050565k.

[325] Journal of Agricultural and Food Chemistry, Milbury PE, Kalt W, Xenobiotic Metabolism and Berry Flavonoids Transport Across the Blood-Brain Barrier, April 14, 2010, vol 58, no 7, 3950-3960, doi:10.1021/jf903529m.

[326] Journal of Agricultural and Food Chemistry, Kalt W, Blumberg JB, McDonald JE, et al. Identification of Anthocyanins in the Liver, Eye, and Brain of Blueberry-fed Pigs, February 13, 2008, vol 56, no 3, 705-712, doi:10.1021/jf071998l.

[327] Journal of Agricultural and Food Chemistry, Milbury PE, Kalt W, Xenobiotic Metabolism and Berry Flavonoids Transport Across the Blood-Brain Barrier, April 14, 2010, vol 58, no 7, 3950-3960, doi:10.1021/jf903529m.

[328] Journal of Agricultural and Food Chemistry, Jing P, Bosmer JA, Schwartz SJ, et al., Structure-Function Relationships of Anthocyanins From Various Anthocyanin-Ric Extracts on the Inhibition of Colon Cancer Cell Growth, Oct 22, 2008, Vol 56(20), 9391-9398, doi:10.1021/jf8005917.

[329] Anti-Cancer agents in Medicinal Chemistry, Katsargyris A, Tampaki EC, Giaginis C, et al., Cranberry as Natural Source of Potential Anti-Cancer Agents: Current Evidence and Future Perspectives, July 2012, 12(6), 619-30, PMID: 22043998.

[330] Current Medicinal Chemistry, Fimognari C, Lenzi M, Hrelia P, Chemoprevention of Cancer by Isothiocyanates and Anthocyanins: Mechanisms of Action and Structure-Activity Relationship, 2008, 15(5), 440-7, PMID:18288999.

[331] Journal of Medicinal Food, Martin KR, Wooden A, Tart Cherry Juice Induces Differential Dose-Dependent Effects on Apoptosis, but not Cellular Proliferation, in MCF-7 Human Breast Cancer Cells, Nov 2012, 15(11), 945-54, doi:10.1089/jmf.2011.0336.

[332] Plant Physiology and Biochemistry, Mazzucato A, Willims D, Bernini R et al., Novel Phenotypes Related to the Breeding of Purple Fruited-Tomatoes and Effect of Peel Extracts on Human Cancer Cell Proliferation, Nov 2013, vol 72, 125-133, doi:10.1016/j.plaphy.2013.05.012.

[333] Frontiers in Aging Neuroscience, Walk Ann M, The Role of Retinol Carotenoids and Age on Neuroelecrtic Indices of Attentional Control Among Early to Middle-Aged Adults, June 9, 2017, doi.org10.3389/fnagi.2017.00183

[334] National Cancer Institute, Cruciferous Vegetables and Cancer Prevention, June 7, 2012. https://www.cancer.gov/about-cancer/causes-prevention/risk/diet/cruciferous-vegetables-fact-sheet.

[335] National Cancer Institute, Cruciferous Vegetables and Cancer Prevention, June 7, 2012. https://www.cancer.gov/about-cancer/causes-prevention/risk/diet/cruciferous-vegetables-fact-sheet.

[336] National Cancer Institute, Cruciferous Vegetables and Cancer Prevention, June 7, 2012. https://www.cancer.gov/about-cancer/causes-prevention/risk/diet/cruciferous-vegetables-fact-sheet.

[337] National Cancer Institute, Cruciferous Vegetables and Cancer Prevention, June 7, 2012. https://www.cancer.gov/about-cancer/causes-prevention/risk/diet/cruciferous-vegetables-fact-sheet.

[338] National Cancer Institute, Cruciferous Vegetables and Cancer Prevention,

June 7, 2012. https://www.cancer.gov/about-cancer/causes-prevention/risk/diet/cruciferous-vegetables-fact-sheet

[339] National Cancer Institute, Cruciferous Vegetables and Cancer Prevention, June 7, 2012. https://www.cancer.gov/about-cancer/causes-prevention/risk/diet/cruciferous-vegetables-fact-sheet

[340] National Cancer Institute, Cruciferous Vegetables and Cancer Prevention, June 7, 2012. https://www.cancer.gov/about-cancer/causes-prevention/risk/diet/cruciferous-vegetables-fact-sheet

[341] Molecular Nutrition and Food Research, Islam S, Akhtar M, Ciavattini A, et al., Use of Dietary Phytochemicals to Target Inflammation, Fibrosis, Proliferation, and Angiogenesis in Uterine Tissues: Promising Options for Prevention and Treatment of Uterine Fibroids?, Aug 2014, 58(8), 1667-1684. doi:10.1002/mnfr.201400134.

[342] Proceedings of the National Academy of Sciences of the United States of America, Bansal T, Alaniz RC, Wood TK, et al. The Bacterial Signal Indole Increases Epithelial-Cell Tight-Junction Resistance and Attenuates Indicators of Inflammation, Jan 5, 2010, vol 107, no 1, 228-233, doi:10.1073/pnas.0906112107.

[343] Inflammopharmacology, Yanaka A, Zhang S, Tauchi M, et al. Role of the nrf-2 Gene in Protection and Repair of Gastric Mucosa Against Oxidative Stress, 2005, 13(1-3):83-90, doi:10.1163/156856005774423863.

[344] Molecular Nutrition and Food Research, Vauzour D, Buonfiglio M, Corona G, et al. Sulforaphane Protects Cortical Neurons Against 5-S-Cysteinyl-Dopamine-Induced Toxicity Through the Activation of ERK1/2,Nrf-2 and the Upregulation of Detoxification Enzymes, April 2010, volume 54, no 4, 532-542, doi:10.1002/mnfr.200900197.

[345] Molecular Nutrition and Food Research, Islam S, Akhtar M, Ciavattini A, et al., Use of Dietary Phytochemicals to Target Inflammation, Fibrosis, Proliferation, and Angiogenesis in Uterine Tissues: Promising Options for Prevention and Treatment of Uterine Fibroids?, Aug 2014, 58(8), 1667-1684. doi:10.1002/mnfr.201400134.

The Sum Is Greater Than the Individual Parts

[346] Journal of Immunology Research, Rodrigo A, Quintero-Fabian S, Lopez-Roa R, et al. Immunomodulation and Anti-inflammatory Effects of Garlic Compounds, April 19, 2015, vol 2015, doi:10.1155/2015/401630.

[347] Journal of Immunology Research, Rodrigo A, Quintero-Fabian S, Lopez-Roa R, et al. Immunomodulation and Anti-inflammatory Effects of Garlic Compounds, April 19, 2015, vol 2015, doi: 10.1155/2015/401630.

[348] Journal of Immunology Research, Rodrigo A, Quintero-Fabian S, Lopez-Roa R, et al. Immunomodulation and Anti-inflammatory Effects of Garlic Compounds, April 19, 2015, vol 2015, doi: 10.1155/2015/401630.

[349] Critical Reviews in Food Science and Nutrition, Butt Masood S, Sultan MT, Butt Mehood S, et al. Garlic: Natures Protection Against Physiological Threats, June 2009, vol 49, no 6, 538-551, doi: 10.1080/10408390802145344.

The Sum Is Greater Than the Individual Parts for All Vegetables

[350] European Journal of Epidemiology, Leenders M, Boshuizen HC, Ferrari P, et al. Fruit and Vegetable Intake and Cause-Specific Mortality in the EPIC Study, Sep 2014, vol 29, no 9, 639-652, doi:10.1007/s10654-014-9945-9.

[351] Lancet, Miller V, Mente A, Dehghan M, et al. Fruit, Vegetable, and Legume

Intake, and Cardiovascular Disease and Deaths in 18 Countries (PURE): a Prospective Cohort Study, Nov 4, 2017, vol 390, no 10107, 2037-2049, doi:10.1016/S0140-6736(17)32253-5.

[352] Lancet, Miller V, Mente A, Dehghan M, et al. Fruit, Vegetable, and Legume Intake, and Cardiovascular Disease and Deaths in 18 Countries (PURE): a Prospective Cohort Study, Nov 4, 2017, vol 390, no 10107, 2037-2049, doi:10.1016/S0140-6736(17)32253-5.

[353] Lancet, GBD 2013 Mortality and Causes of Death Collaborators, Global, Regional, and National Age-Sex Specific All-Cause and Cause-Specific Mortality for 240 Causes of Death, 1990-2013: a Systemic Analysis for the Global Burden of Disease Study 2013, Jan 10, 2015, vol 385, no 9963, 117-171, doi:10.1016/S0140-6736(14)61682-2.

[354] UN General Assembly. United Nations High-Level Meeting on Noncommunicable Disease Prevention and Control. NCD Summit to Shape the International Agenda New York, 2011, http://www.who.int/nmh/events/un_ncd_summit2011/en/.

[355] UN General Assembly. United Nations High-Level Meeting on Noncommunicable Disease Prevention and Control. NCD Summit to Shape the International Agenda New York, 2011, http://www.who.int/nmh/events/un_ncd_summit2011/en/.

[356] UN General Assembly. United Nations High-Level Meeting on Noncommunicable Disease Prevention and Control. NCD Summit to Shape the International Agenda New York, 2011, http://www.who.int/nmh/events/un_ncd_summit2011/en/.

What's the Deal With Short-Chain Fatty Acids?

[357] Nature Communications, Macia L, Tan J, Vieira AT, et al. Metabolite-Sensing Receptors GPR43 and GPR109A Facilitate Dietary Fibre-Induced Gut Homeostasis Through Regulation of the Inflammasome, Apr 1, 2015, vol 6, 6734, doi:10.1038/ncomms7734.

[358] Immunity, Singh N, Gurav A, Sivaprakasam S, et al. Activation of Gpr109a Receptor for Niacin and the Commensal Metabolite Butyrate, Suppresses Colonic Inflammation and Carcinogenesis, Jan 16, 2014, vol 40, no 1, 128-139, doi:10.1016/j.immuni.2013.12.007.

[359] Cell Metabolism, Donohoe DR, Garge N, Zhang X, et al. The Microbiome and Butyrate Regulate Energy Metabolism and Autophagy in the Mammalian Colon, May 4, 2011, vol 13, no 5, 517-526, doi:10.1016/j.cmet.2011.02.018.

[360] Proceedings of the National Academy of Sciences of the United States of America, Raqib R, Sarker P, Bergman P, et al. Improved Outcome in Shigellosis Associated with Butyrate Induction of an Endogenous Peptide Antibiotic, Jun 13, 2006, vol 103, no 24, 9178-9183, doi:10.1073/pnas.0602888103.

[361] Scientific Reports, Pozuelo M, Panda S, Santiago A, et al. Reduction of Butyrate- and Methane-Producing Microorganisms in Patients with Irritable Bowel Syndrome, 2015, vol 5, 12693, doi:10.1038/srep12693.

[362] Inflammatory Bowel Disease, Menzel T, Luhrs H, Zirlik S, et al. Butyrate Inhibits Leukocyte Adhesion to Endothelial Cells via Modulation of VCAM-1, Mar 2004, vol 10, no 2, 122-128, doi:10.1097/00054725-200403000-00010.

[363] Scientific Reports, Ji J, Shu D, Zheng M, et al. Microbial Metabolite Butyrate Facilitates M2 Macrophage Polarization and Function, 2016, vol6, 24838, doi:10.1038/srep24838.

[364] Scientific Reports, Geirnaert A, Calatayud M, Grootaert C, et al. Butyrate-Producing Bacteria Supplemented in vitro to Crohn's Disease Patient Microbiota Increased Butyrate Production and Enhanced Intestinal Epithelial Barrier

Integrity, 2017, vol 7, 11450, doi:10.1038/s41598-017-11734-8.
[365] Nutrition in Clinical Practice: Official Publication of the American Society for Parenteral and Enteral Nutrition, Roy CC, Kien CL, Bouthillier L, et al. Aug 2006, vol 21, no 4, 351-366, doi:10.1177/0115426506021004351.
[366] Cell, Clemente JC, Ursell LK, Parfrey LW, et al. The Impact of the Gut Microbiota on Human Health: an Integrative View, Mar 16, 2012, vol 148, no 6, doi:10.1016/j.cell.2012,01.035.
[367] Proceedings of the National Academy of Sciences of the United States of America, Greenblum S, Turnbaugh PJ, Borenstein E, Metagenomic Systems Biology of the Human Gut Microbiome Reveals Topological Shifts Associated with Obesity and Inflammatory Bowel Disease, Jan 10, 2012, vol 109, no 2, 594-595, doi:10.1073/pnas.1116053109.
[368] Nature, Maslowski KM, Vieira AT, Ng A, et al. Regulation of Inflammatory Responses by Gut Microbiota and Chemoattractant Receptor GPR43, Oct 29, 2009, vol 461, no 7268, 1282-1286, doi:10.1038/nature08530.
[369] Nature, Maslowski KM, Vieira AT, Ng A, et al. Regulation of Inflammatory Responses by Gut Microbiota and Chemoattractant Receptor GPR43, Oct 29, 2009, vol 461, no 7268, 1282-1286, doi:10.1038/nature08530.
[370] Nature, Maslowski KM, Vieira AT, Ng A, et al. Regulation of Inflammatory Responses by Gut Microbiota and Chemoattractant Receptor GPR43, Oct 29, 2009, vol 461, no 7268, 1282-1286, doi:10.1038/nature08530.
[371] Scientific Reports, Geirnaert A, Calatayud M, Grootaert C, et al. Butyrate-Producing Bacteria Supplemented in vitro to Crohn's Disease Patient Microbiota Increased Butyrate Production and Enhanced Intestinal Epithelial Barrier Integrity, 2017, vol 7, 11450, doi:10.1038/s41598-017-11734-8.
[372] The Proceedings of the Nutrition Society, Malcomson FC, Willis ND, Mathers JC, Is Resistant Starch Protective Against Coloretal Cancer via Modulation of the WNT Signaling Pathway?, Aug 2015, vol 74, no 3, 282-291, doi:10.1017/S002966511500004x.
[373] The Proceedings of the Nutrition Society, Malcomson FC, Willis ND, Mathers JC, Is Resistant Starch Protective Against Coloretal Cancer via Modulation of the WNT Signaling Pathway?, Aug 2015, vol 74, no 3, 282-291, doi:10.1017/S002966511500004x.
[374] Molecular Endocrinology, Clarke G, Stilling RM, Kennedy PJ, et al. Minireview: Gut Microbiota: The Neglected Endocrine Organ, Aug 2014, vol 28, no 8, 1221-1238, doi:10.1210/me.2014-1108.
[375] Science Translational Medicine, Braniste V, Al-Asmakh M, Kowal C, et al. The Gut Microbiota Influences Blood-Brain Barrier Permeability in Mice, Nov 19, 2014, vol 6, no 263, 263ra158, doi:10.1126/scitranslmed.3009759.
[376] Aluko RE, Functional Foods and Nutraceuticals, Bioactive Lipids, New York Springer Science Business Media, 2012, 23-36.
[377] The Journal of Nutrition, Hara H, Haga S, Aoyama Y, et al. Short-Chain Fatty Acids Suppress Cholesterol Synthesis in Rat Liver and Intestine, May 1999, vol 129, no 5, 942-948, doi:10.1093/jn/129.5.942.
[378] Microbiome, Hoyles L, Snelling T, Umm-Kulthum U, et al. Microbiome-Host Systems Interactions: Protective Effects of Propionate Upon the Blood-Brain Barrier, Mar 21, 2018, vol 6, 55, doi:10.1186/s40168-018-0439-y
[379] European Spine Journal: Official Publication of the European Spine Society, the European Spinal Deformity Society, and the European Section of the Cervical Spine Research Society, Nagashima H, Morio Y, Meshitsuka S, et al. High-Resolution Nuclear Magnetic Resonance Spectroscopic Study of Metabolites in the Cerebrospinal Fluid of Patients with Cervical Myelopathy and Lumbar Radiculopathy, Aug 2010, vol 19, no 8, 1363-1368,doi:10.1007/s00586-010-1453-3.

[380] Journal of Cerebral Blood Flow and Metabolism: Official of the International Society of Cerebral Blood Flow and Metabolism, Wyss MT, Magistretti PJ, Buck A, et al. Labeled Acetate as a Marker of Astrocytic Metabolism, Aug 2011, vol 31 no 8, 1668-1674, doi:10.1038/jcbfm.2011.84.

[381] Nature Communications, Frost G, Sleeth ML, Sahuri-Arisoylu M, et al. The Short-Chain Fatty Acid Acetate Reduces Appetite via a Central Homeostatic Mechanism, Apr 29, 2014, vol 5, 3611, doi:10.1038.ncomms4611.

[382] Mucosal Immunology, Wu W, Sun M, Chen F, et al. Microbiota Metabolite Short-Chain Fatty Acid Acetate Promotes Intestinal IgA Response to Microbiota Which is Mediated by GPR43, Jul 2017, vol 10, no 4, 946-956, doi:10.1038/mi.2016.114.

[383] Immunological Reviews, Gutzeit C, Magri G, Cerutti A, Intestinal IgA Production and its Role in Host-Microbe Interaction, Jun 19, 2014, vol 260, no 1, 76-85, doi:10.1111/imr.12189.

[384] Hormone and Metabolic Research, Roshanravan N, Mahdavi R, Alizadeh E, et al. Effect of Butyrate and Inulin Supplementation on Glycemic Status, Lipid Profile and Glucagon-Like eptide 1 Level in Patients with Type 2 Diabetes: A Randomized Double-Blind, Placebo-Controlled Trail, Nov 2017, vol 49, no 11, 886-891, doi:10.1055/s-0043-119089.

[385] The Proceedings of the Nutrition Society, Fava F, Rizetto L, Tuohy KM, Gut Microbiota and Health: Connecting Actors Across the Metabolic System, Dec 18, 2018, 1-12, doi:10.1017/S0029665118002719.

[386] Current Opinion in Clinical Nutrition and Metabolic Care, Ryan PM, Ross RP, Fitzgerald GF, et al. Functional Food Addressing Heart Health: do we Have to Target the Gut Microbiota?, Nov 2015, vol 18, no 6, doi:10.1097/MCO.0000000000000224.

[387] Microbial Biotechnology, Xu H, Wang X, Feng W, et al, The gut Microbiota and its Interactions with Cardiovascular Disease, Jan 26, 2020, doi:10.1111/1751-7915.13524.

[388] Expert Review of Endocrinology & Metabolism, Warmbrunn MV, Herrema H, Aron-Wisnewsky J, et al. Gut Microbiota: a Promising Target Against Cardiometabolic Diseases, Jan 2020, vol 15, no 1, 13-27, doi:10.1080/17446651.2020.1720511.

[389] Journal of the American College of Cardiology, Tang WHW, Backhed F, Landmesser U, et al. Intestinal Microbiota in Cardiovascular Health and Disease: JACC State-of-the-Art Review, Apr 30, 2019, vol 73, no 16, 2089-2105, doi:10.1016/j.jacc.2019.03.024.

[390] US Department of Agriculture: Agricultural Research Service, What We Eat in America: Nutrient Intakes From Food by Gender and age, National Health and Nutrition Examination Survey (NHANES) 2009-2010, www.ars.usda.gov/Sp2userfiles/Place/12355000/Pdf/0910/Table_1_Nin_Gen_0 9.Pdf.

[391] Circulation, Lloyd-Jones DM, Hong Y, Labarthe D, et al. Defining and Setting National Goals for Cardiovascular Health Promotion and Disease Reduction: the American Heart Association's Strategic Impact Goal Through 2020 and Beyond, Feb 2, 2010, vol 121, no 4, 586-613, doi:10.1161/CIRCULATIONAHA.109.192703.

[392] Circulation, Lloyd-Jones DM, Hong Y, Labarthe D, et al. Defining and Setting National Goals for Cardiovascular Health Promotion and Disease Reduction: the American Heart Association's Strategic Impact Goal Through 2020 and Beyond, Feb 2, 2010, vol 121, no 4, 586-613, doi:10.1161/CIRCULATIONAHA.109.192703.

[393] Journal of Cardiovascular Pharmacology, Yamagata K, Yamori Y, Inhibition of Endothelial Dysfunction by Dietary Flavonoids and Preventive Effects Against

Cardiovascular Disease, Jan 2020, vol 75, no 1, 1-9, doi:10.1097/FJC.0000000000000757.

[394] Journal of the American Heart Association, Sotos-Prieto M, Mattel J, Cook N, et al. Association Between a 20-Year Cardiovascular Disease Risk Score Based on Modifiable Lifestyles and Total and Cause-Specific Mortality Among US Men and Women, Nov 6, 2018, vol 7, no 21, doi:10.1161/JAHA.118.010052.

[395] Current Nutrition Reports, Chambers ES, Preston T, Frost G, et al. Role of Gut Microbiota-Generated Short-Chain Fatty Acids in Metabolic and Cardiovascular Health, Dec 2018, vol 7, no 4, 198-206, doi:10.1007/s13668-018-0248-8.

[396] Ciculation Kaye DM, Shihata W, Jama HA, et al. Deficiency of Prebiotic Fibre and Insufficient Signalling Through Gut Metabolite Sensing Receptors Leads to Cardiovascular Disease, Feb 25, 2020, doi:10.1161/CIRCULATIONAHA.119.043081.

[397] The British Journal of Nutrition, Buil-Cosiales P, Toledo E, Salas-Salvado J, et al. Association Between Dietary Fibre Intake and Fruit, Vegetable or Whole-Grain Consumption and the Risk of CVD: Results From the PREvencion con DIeta MEDiterranea (PREMED) Trial, Aug 2016, vol 116, no 3, 534-546, doi:10.1017/S0007114516002099.

[398] Current Nutrition Reports, Chambers ES, Preston T, Frost G, et al. Role of Gut Microbiota-Generated Short-Chain Fatty Acids in Metabolic and Cardiovascular Health, Dec 2018, vol 7, no 4, 198-206, doi:10.1007/s13668-018-0248-8.

[399] The Proceedings of the Nutrition Society, Fava F, Rizetto L, Tuohy KM, Gut Microbiota and Health: Connecting Actors Across the Metabolic System, Dec 18, 2018, 1-12, doi:10.1017/S0029665118002719.

[400] Diabetes & Metabolic Syndrome, Bolori P, Setaysh L, Rasaei N, et al. Adherence to a Healthy Plant Diet may Reduce Inflammatory Factors in Obese and Overweight Women-a Cross-Sectional Study, Jul-Aug 2019, vol 13 no 4, 2795-2802, doi:10.1016/j.dsx.2019.07.019.

[401] Nutrients, Okouchi R, E S, Yamamoto K, et al. Simultaneous Intake of Euglena Gracilis and Vegetables Exerts Synergistic Anti-Obesity and Anti-Inflammatory Effects by modulating the Gut Microbiota on Diet-Induced Obese Mice, Jan 21, 2019, vol 11, no 1, doi:10.3390/nu11010204.

[402] The Proceedings of the Nutrition Society, Fava F, Rizetto L, Tuohy KM, Gut Microbiota and Health: Connecting Actors Across the Metabolic System, Dec 18, 2018, 1-12, doi:10.1017/S0029665118002719.

[403] Journal of Diabetes Investigation, Wang PU, Fang JC, Gao ZH, et al. Higher Intake of Fruits, Vegetables or their Fiber Reduces the Risk of Type 2 Diabetes: A Meta-Analysis, Jan 2016, vol 7, no 156-69, doi:10.1111/jdi.12376.

[404] The Journal of Nutrition, Aie HB, Ley SH, Rosner B, et al. High Fiber and Low Starch Intakes are Associated with Circulating Intermediate Biomarkers of Type 2 Diabetes Among Women, Feb 2016, vol 146, no 2, 306-317, doi:10.3945/jn.115.219915.

[405] Diabetologia, InterAct Consortium, Kuijsten A, Aune D, Schulze MB, et al. Dietary Fibre and Incidence of Type 2 Diabetes in Eight European Countries: the EPIC-InterAct Study and a Meta-Analysis of Prospective Studies, Jul 2015, vol 58, no 7, 1394-1408, doi:10.1007/s00125-015-3585-9.

Plants Used as Pharmaceuticals

[406] Dansk Medicinhistorisk Arbog, Norn S, Kruse PR, (Cardiac Glycosides: From Ancient History Through Withering's Foxglove to Endogenous Cardiac

Glycosides), 2004, 119-132, PMID:15685783.
[407] https://www.pharmacognosy.us/what-is-pharmacognosy/the-history-of-the-asp/
[408] Journal of Natural Products, Newman D, Cragg G, Natural Products as Sources of New Drugs Over the 30 Years From 1981-2010, March 23, 2012, vol 75,no 3, 311-335, doi:10.1021/np200906s.
[409] Journal of Adavnced Pharamaceutical Technology & Research, Veeresham C, Natural products Deirved From Plants as a Source of Drugs, Oct-Dec 2012, vol 3, no 4, 200-201, doi:10.4103/2231-4040.104709.
[410] Environmental Health Perspectives, Fabricant DS, Farnsworth NR, The Value of Plants Used in Traditional Medicine for Drug Discovery, March 2001, vol 109, supp 1, 69-75, doi:10.1289/ehp.01109s169.
[411] Environmental Health Perspectives, Fabricant DS, Farnsworth NR, The Value of Plants Used in Traditional Medicine for Drug Discovery, March 2001, vol 109, supp 1, 69-75, doi:10.1289/ehp.01109s169.
[412] Journal of Natural Products, Newman DJ, Cragg GM, Natural Products as Sources of New Drugs Over the 30 Years From 1981 to2010, Mar 23, 2012, vol 75, no 3, 311-335, doi:10.1021/np200906s.
[413] Journal of Natural Products, Newman DJ, Cragg GM, Natural Products as Sources of New Drugs From 1981 to2014, Mar 25, 2016, vol 79, no 3, 629-661, doi:10.1021/acs.jnatprod.5b0155.
[414] Journal of Natural Products, Newman DJ, Cragg GM, Natural Products as Sources of New Drugs From 1981 to2014, Mar 25, 2016, vol 79, no 3, 629-661, doi:10.1021/acs.jnatprod.5b0155.
[415] Journal of Natural Products, Newman DJ, Cragg GM, Natural Products as Sources of New Drugs From 1981 to2014, Mar 25, 2016, vol 79, no 3, 629-661, doi:10.1021/acs.jnatprod.5b0155.
[416]Journal of Natural Products, Newman D, Cragg G, Natural Products as Sources of New Drugs Over the 30 Years From 1981-2010, March 23, 2012, vol 75,no 3, 311-335, doi:10.1021/np200906s.
[417] Journal of Natural Products, Newman D, Cragg G, Natural Products as Sources of New Drugs Over the 30 Years From 1981-2010, March 23, 2012, vol 75,no 3, 311-335, doi:10.1021/np200906s.
[418] Journal of Natural Products, Newman D, Cragg G, Natural Products as Sources of New Drugs Over the 30 Years From 1981-2010, March 23, 2012, vol 75,no 3, 311-335, doi:10.1021/np200906s.
[419] Microbiology and Molecular Biology Reviews, Hardoim PR, van Overbeek LS, Berg G, et al. The Hidden World Within Plants: Ecological and Evolutionary Considerations for Defining Functioning of Microbial Endophytes, Sep 2015, vol 79, no 3, 293-320, doi:10.1128/MMBR.00050-14.
[420] Journal of Natural Products, Leslie Gunatilaka AA, Natural Products From Plant-Associated Microorganisms: Distribution, Structural Diversity, Bioactivity, and Implications of Their Occurrence, Mar 2006, vol 69, no 3, 509-526, doi:10.1021/np058128n.
[421] Microbiology and Molecular Biology Reviews, Strobel G, Daisy B, Bioprospecting for Microbial Endophytes and Their Natural Products, Dec 2003, vol 67, no 4, 491-502, doi:10.1128/MMBR.67.4.491-502.2003.
[422] Journal of Natural Products, Strobel G, Daisy B, Castillo U, et a. Natural Products From Endophytic Microorganisms, Feb 2004, vol 67, no 2, 257-268. Doi:10.1021/np030397v.
[423] Natural Products Communications, Verma VC, Kharwar RN, Strobel GA, Chemical and Functional diversity of Natural Products From Plant Associated Endophytic Fungi, Nov 2009. Vol 4, no 11, 1511-1532, PMID:19967984.
[424] Natural Product Reports, Tan RX, Zou WX, Endophytes: a Rich Source of

Functional Metabolites, Aug 2001, vol 18, no 4, 448-459.
Doi:10.1039/b100918o.
[425] Applied Microbiology and Biotechnology, Aly AH, Debbab A, Proksch P, Fungal Endophytes: Unique Plant Inhabitants with Great Promises, Jun 2011, vol 90, no 6, 1829-1845, doi:10.1007/s00253-011-3270-y.
[426] Fungal Diversity, Aly AH, Debbab A, Kjer J, et al. Fungal Endophytes From Higher Plants: a Profile Source of Phytochemicals and Other Bioactive Natural Products, 2010, vol 41, 1-16, doi:10.1007/s13225-010-0034-4.
[427] Natural Product Reports, Zhang HW, Song YC, Tan RX, Biology and Chemistry of Endophytes, Oct 2006, vol 23, no 5, 753-771, doi:10.1039b609472b.

Let's Sum This Up
[428] Cancer Facts and Figures 2014,
https://www.cancer.org/content/dam/cancer-org/research/cancer-facts-and-statistics/annual-cancer-facts-and-figures/2014/cancer-facts-and-figures-2014.pdf

Made in the USA
Las Vegas, NV
19 October 2021